THE
sexy
years

ALSO BY SUZANNE SOMERS

Touch Me

Keeping Secrets

Wednesday's Children

Suzanne Somers' Eat Great, Lose Weight

Suzanne Somers' Get Skinny on Fabulous Food

After the Fall

Suzanne Somers' 365 Ways to Change Your Life

Suzanne Somers' Eat, Cheat, and Melt the Fat Away

Somersize Desserts

Suzanne Somers' Fast and Easy

THE
sexy
years

DISCOVER THE HORMONE CONNECTION:

THE SECRET TO FABULOUS SEX, GREAT HEALTH,

AND VITALITY, FOR WOMEN AND MEN

SUZANNE SOMERS

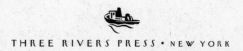

THREE RIVERS PRESS • NEW YORK

Copyright © 2004 by Suzanne Somers
Foreword copyright © 2004 by Robert A. Greene, M.D., FACOG

Published in the United States by Three Rivers Press
an imprint of the Crown Publishing Group,
a division of Random House, Inc., New York
www.crownpublishing.com

THREE RIVERS PRESS and the tugboat design are registered trademarks
of Random House, Inc.

Originally published in hardcover in the United States by Crown Publishers,
an imprint of the Crown Publishing Group, a division of Random House, Inc.,
New York

Printed in the United States of America

DESIGN BY ELINA D. NUDELMAN

Library of Congress Cataloging-in-Publication Data
Somers, Suzanne, 1946–
The sexy years : discover the hormone connection : the secret to fabulous sex,
great health, and vitality, for women and men / Suzanne Somers.—1st ed.
1. Hormones—Popular works.   2. Middle aged women—Health and hygiene—
Popular works.   3. Middle aged men—Health and hygiene—Popular works.
4. Somers, Suzanne, 1946—Health.   I. Title.
QP571.S65   2004
613'.0434—dc22   2003023601

ISBN 1-4000-8157-2

10 9 8 7 6 5 4 3 2 1

First Paperback Edition

TO MY HUSBAND, ALAN

You turn me on!

ACKNOWLEDGMENTS

I feel so blessed to have such talented people around me.

Once again, my editor, Kristin Kiser, was an enormous help to me in this massive undertaking. When I would get overwhelmed, she would be there to help me through the maze. Thank you, Kristin.

My agent, Al Lowman, is the greatest agent in the literary world. No one is better at it than Al. He is there from the very beginning to the very last detail. We've done so many books together that I have lost count. I only know I wouldn't do a book without you. Thank you, Al. I love you.

My husband, Alan Hamel, takes care of everything so all I have to do is keep on writing. I am so lucky to have Alan running the show, as they say. I'm crazy in love with you, Alan.

Sandi Mendelson and Judy Hilsinger are fantastic press agents. They are nurturing and creative simultaneously. Doesn't matter how great a book you write—if the public doesn't know about it, nothing happens. When Sandi and Judy do the press on one of my books, everybody knows about it. You two are the greatest. Thank you so much.

My lawyer Marc Chamlin, thank you once again.

My lawyer Martin Hahn, thank you.

And to my fabulous team at Crown Publishing . . .

Jenny Frost, president and publisher of Crown, this is our first book together, and what a way to start. You have been enthusiastic about this idea from the very beginning. Your getting behind this project has had a tremendous positive impact. Thank you.

Steve Ross, my publisher at Crown, you are always in my corner, but for this one even a little more so. Your enthusiasm has been catching and now everyone is feeling it. I couldn't ask for more. Thank you so much.

Philip Patrick, director of marketing, you are wonderful to work with. You have done so much front work on this project that everyone you are working with can't wait to get this book. Thanks for all the advance excitement.

Tina Constable, director of publicity, you are a hard-working professional and so talented and creative. I have enjoyed our relationship over the years. Thanks so much for all your input and enthusiasm.

Mary Schuck, jacket designer, I love this cover. Maybe the favorite of all my books. Thank you. Just beautiful.

Elina Nudelman, interior designer. I love it. Thank you.

Amy Boorstein, Camille Smith, Leta Evanthes, Ellen Rubinstein, thanks to all of you for all your input and hard work.

Sona Vogel, you did a great job copyediting this difficult manuscript. I was impressed with your abilities, and I learned new things through your corrections. Thank you.

Thanks to Caroline Somers, my daughter-in-law, for that great idea. It was just what I needed to hear at that moment. You know how much I love you.

And Marsha Yanchuck, my assistant of twenty-six years, thank you for reading and rereading each and every draft and giving me suggestions and for your expertise on grammar and punctuation. You have helped me through so many books, but this one in particular was the most tedious. Thank you. You are more than my loyal assistant—you are my family and I love you dearly.

And now to my great doctors, who gave so freely of themselves for this book. These doctors, all of whom are cutting-edge and forward-thinking, are going to change the direction of medicine. They are pioneers who are willing to stick their necks out to get the latest information out to the public, regardless of the risks. Thank you all for allowing me to offer you a platform.

Dr. Diana Schwarzbein, you are the first doctor I found to specialize in this subject, and because of you my life has changed for the better. You have been invaluable to me as a teacher and a doctor. Thank you for the constant barrage of information you continue to send me. Words cannot express my appreciation.

Dr. Eugene Shippen, you are brilliant. Finally there is a doctor to help men through this least understood passage of male menopause. Thank you for all your help and input. I am deeply indebted to you.

Dr. Michael Galitzer, you are an absolute joy to work with and so informed and educated on this subject. Already you have helped so many people I have sent to you. Thank you for giving so freely of yourself and your knowledge.

Dr. Uzzi Reiss, you are a wonderful, compassionate, and knowledgeable doctor who is helping women more than you will ever know. Thank you for your time and information. I appreciate everything you have done for me and this project.

Dr. Laura Berman, you are an absolute font of information on this subject. Thank you for your knowledge and expertise in this area. A lot of women are going to be helped by your chapter.

Dr. Jennifer Berman, thank you for giving so freely of your knowledge. I came away impressed and grateful for your input. I also learned a lot.

Dr. Robert Greene, thank you for your beautiful foreword, your cutting-edge insights, and your profound enthusiasm for this project.

And finally, my ladies: Karen, Athena, Rita, Patricia, Eve, Marta, and my sister, Maureen Gilmartin. Each of you gave of yourselves with honesty and sincerity. You allowed me to crawl inside your heads for a few pages. You are living this passage, and your candor and wisdom are thrilling. I am grateful to all of you for your honesty and insights.

Thank you to everyone who helped me with this project. I am grateful and honored to be able to bring this exciting new information to the American public, but I could not have done it without all of you.

CONTENTS

PART III
Life on Your Own Terms

PART IV
The Male Menopause

PART V

Beating the Clock

PART VI

Living an Authentic Life

At fifty, you get
the face you deserve.

—COCO CHANEL

FOREWORD

BY ROBERT A. GREENE, M.D., FACOG

I am a reproductive endocrinologist. That means that after becoming a board-certified ob-gyn, I continued my training to become a specialist in identifying and treating hormone-related problems such as those associated with infertility, menopause, developmental problems, and premenstrual syndrome. During the last decade, I have continued to perform research in this field and apply what I learn on a daily basis to the patients whom I provide care for. Developing an understanding of the way hormones affect the brain is truly the key to lifelong health and wellness.

As a reproductive endocrinologist, my primary focus is on the sex hormones: estrogen, progesterone, and testosterone. Women today are heavily influenced by the marketing of "natural" hormones. But what do we mean by "natural"? There is no unified definition of the term "natural hormones." Natural means different things to different people. To some people natural means that it comes from natural sources. To others, it means biologically identical to what the body normally produces. That's the definition that Suzanne and I have used during our discussions of this topic. The confusion about this terminology dates back to 1941 when Russell Marker first synthesized progesterone from the wild yam, *Dioscorea*. To this day, many companies sell "natural yam extracts" as alternatives to hormones. Unfortunately, they fail to inform consumers that their bodies simply do not have the ability to convert this plant extract to an active, usable hormone, like what is accomplished in a laboratory.

The sex hormones are able to work in the body through specific receptors—imagine a lock-and-key system. Any given part of the human body has to have the proper receptor, or lock, for a specific hormone to have an effect. There are at least two different types of estrogen receptors in the body. These receptors vary in concentration in different parts of the body, which means the estrogen potency varies as well according to its ability to occupy the receptors. Understanding these variations is crucial in order to stabilize hormone disturbances that occur throughout your life because, if you're a woman, your hormone levels are shifting, sometimes on a daily basis. Individualized regimens from your doctor provide specific treatment so that each woman can maintain optimal hormonal levels and feel her best. The word *balance* is the most important goal in maintaining a state of equilibrium.

Establishing that perfect balance is challenging; it can almost seem daunting to take the time to learn the myriad functions of the abundant hormones that direct our daily activities. Many clinicians get comfortable with one or two preparations and try to fit everybody into a "one size fits all." This just doesn't work. It might satisfy about 15 percent of the people, but the remaining 85 percent struggle with unnecessary discomfort. Achieving and maintaining your unique hormonal balance is very important, and demanding nothing less from your doctor will empower you to guide your own sense of well-being.

As a doctor and an advocate for women with hormonal imbalances, I'm frustrated. I do about 120 lectures a year in different parts of the country, primarily geared toward empathetic clinicians interested in improving health care. But we are increasingly forced to spend less and less time with our patients due to insurance company dictates. We also must stay apprised of current research findings, which are frequently misinterpreted. These constraints create barriers to communication, difficult for some in the best of circumstances. Patients are frustrated. Today's women want more than a diagnosis from their doctors. It is not an uncommon complaint of women that they feel that their physician marginalizes their complaints with tired comments: "Oh, you're just imagining things," or "You just need to accept that as a natural part of aging." This is not the kind of response a male patient would typically receive, and it's time we even the playing field. We all want to feel good and we all deserve to feel good. Physicians must recognize that their patients face new challenges and will fight to be heard, and they must respond effectively to their patients' demands.

In the absence of satisfactory health care, a schism develops when women transition into the postreproductive years. Some gain weight and can't figure out why; others might find they are suddenly difficult to get along with. These are just a few of many problems that can result because of the hormonal imbalances that occur over a woman's lifetime, compromising quality of life. Many women tell me that they know their moods are unpredictable, but in most cases they don't have any control over the chemical changes causing these mood shifts. They can't sleep, they're hot, then they are cold, they are tired all day; these are also related to chemical changes in the brain. It is true suffering. The quality of life many of these women enjoyed up until this "passage" into the postreproductive years is suddenly gone. There is a sense of betrayal. I applaud Suzanne Somers' attempt to bridge this communication gap so that women may enjoy continued wellness throughout their lives.

Suzanne asked me why I thought middle-aged men often leave their middle-aged wives. I don't believe it is because middle-aged women don't look good. The reality is women look better now at middle age than they've ever looked before because they know how to take better care of themselves. I fear that some men leave their relationships because they don't understand the effects of this hormonal passage into menopause. They don't have anything in their own physiology to compare it to. Worse yet, women are often told to "tough it out," as if it would be antifeminist to insist on continued wellness. Add to all this the zeroing out of the sex drive, and after a while some men may wind up saying, "What do I need this for?" We at least owe these couples an explanation of the physiological changes associated with hormone withdrawal in order to validate the problems that they may experience. This knowledge can provide a tremendous amount of psychological relief.

My interest in hormonal fluctuations led me to a specific research niche more than ten years ago. Since then my research has been focused on how hormones affect the brain. The adult brain, with all its wonderful and amazing qualities, simply doesn't reach its potential in the absence of normal adult hormone levels. Once you fully appreciate that fact, it is easy to understand the consequences that result if you take those same hormones away—things start to go haywire. Most of my research has been focused on all the different nuances and subtleties of why and how the hormone-brain relationship works; but the bottom line is, you don't maintain your full capabilities if your brain is no longer exposed to the hormone balance it is accustomed to. In the end, women want to make sure they have their brain working optimally, especially since they're living longer than ever before. One of the obstacles that they often face, however, is an apprehension of cancer.

A fear of breast cancer is almost rampant in our society, and my concern is that it clouds our judgment. Cancer is scary. But let's put that fear into perspective, especially in comparison to the brain. Data from various studies show us that for 1,000 women on HRT for ten years, about six additional breast cancers are diagnosed. By comparison, other studies predict that these same 1,000 women taking estrogen would result in about 240 fewer cases of Alzheimer's disease. When you consider that 80 to 90 percent of breast cancers are curable today and there's no cure for Alzheimer's disease, it is easy to realize that at the very least women should be properly informed of all potential benefits of hormone therapy, including healthy aging of the brain. The connection between loss of estrogen and Alzheimer's disease is widely accepted among brain scientists, yet the more general medical community is long overdue in acknowledging this connection. Even more important is for health care practitioners to communicate this information to their patients, which will prevent women from looking to the news media for guidance in health matters, where information is often sensationalized, inaccurate, and should not be generalized to all women. For instance, the Women's Health Initiative Memory Study (WHIMS) came out recently suggesting that estrogen increased dementia, but the average age of the women in that study was nearly seventy-three! The participants were also free of symptoms like hot flashes, night sweats, and mood changes. The age of the study participants was not highlighted in the popular press when they reported this finding, however. If you actually look at the data, the percentage of women who developed Alzheimer's disease was less if they were on hormone therapy (50.0 percent) than if they weren't (57.1 percent). This is a clear-cut case of the irresponsible exploitation of data to scare rather than inform. Whether we blame the scientists interviewed or the reporters is irrelevant—the target audience suffers needlessly.

Regrettably, today's health care decisions are often driven by preconception and assumption. There is a presumed relationship between estrogen and breast cancer, but once upon a time the first treatments given to women with breast cancer were high-dose estrogen therapy, and a significant percentage of women who were treated responded. The belief that estrogen is a carcinogen simply is not supported by well-designed studies or biological plausibility. Did you know that in the third trimester of pregnancy, a woman's hormone output is equal to about ninety-nine years' worth of menopausal doses of hormone replacement? Yet breast cancer is fairly uncommon during the reproductive years. Recently, one of the best-designed studies of women with some of the most common gene mutations associated with breast and ovarian cancer— BRCA1 and BRCA2—found that pregnancy was actually protective against these cancers! They also found that women who started menstruating earlier were not at higher risk despite a greater lifetime exposure to hormones. Yet the same scientists involved in this study were quoted in the *New York Times* (October 24, 2003) as supporting the removal of healthy breasts and ovaries of women with these gene mutations. I have examined the findings of many research studies and it is my belief that HRT is unlikely to be a cause of cancer; it's more likely that hormone therapy promotes the growth of existing tumors. The fear of cancer is legitimate, but it warrants a rational response.

Women come to me out of frustration. Some travel five or six hours to get to my office, which is a shame, but this is an act of desperation to receive treatment options explained in rational terms. For example, one female patient of mine participating in a study on testosterone replacement recently conducted an interview for the FDA. When asked what she would do if the hormone preparation she was taking wasn't approved, she broke into tears. She said, "I can't go back to living that way. I've been given back my life; you can't tell me it might not be approved!" It was tragic to see this spontaneous display of emotion, because you know she really meant it. I hope the FDA begins listening to these answers when they ask questions of study participants.

I believe that in the next decade replacing and rebalancing hormones lost in the aging process will become the standard of care. And not just for women, but for men as well. Until recently, the male menopause (andropause) has been almost completely ignored and men have suffered because of it. Androgen deficiency is real and can be treated. Most men live out their more gradual decline of hormone production in silence, because they feel it is an admission that they are no longer "virile" or "male." The greatest loss that they experience is fatigue and lack of energy as a result of muscle wasting and changes in their brain functioning. I have been fortunate to write articles for and act as a consultant to the International Society for the Study of the Aging Male. We are beginning to understand the role of HRT to restore the male quality of life. In 2002, the Endocrine Society, which is comprised primarily of internal medicine endocrinologists, held a symposium to present guidelines on testosterone replacement for men. This was a very bold step forward in acknowledging the impact on men's quality of life. Ironically, they have not openly embraced a comparable policy for women. Keep in mind that testosterone is no less tenuously linked to prostate cancer than estrogen is to breast cancer.

As doctors we have to listen to our patients. No one can under-stand a person's individual needs as well as that person. There is a new focus on improving quality of life. We need to empower peo-ple, men *and* women, to recognize the symptoms of "too much or too little"—in other words, the symptoms of hormone imbalance. In this way the patient will have sufficient information to choose the appropriate treatment for long-term health and well-being based upon this growing knowledge and understanding of the hormone-brain connection.

Today's patient and provider must form a partnership. Commu-nication in medicine still often struggles with what I call the pater-nalistic style of delivery of health care. Instead of telling their patients what to do, care providers must discuss today's informa-tion openly. If they do not, then demand it; you will be heard. We have a very consumer-driven market, and the paternalistic doctors, some of whom are women, need to understand that. Women seek-ing answers will identify those doctors who are willing to listen to them and then explain their options with full disclosure of risks and benefits. The successful health care providers of the future will encourage thoughtful dialogue through open channels of commu-nication.

It's taken years for the medical community to catch up with peo-ple like Suzanne Somers, who along with several others have been pioneers in equating the insulin connection with weight gain. At first these theories were disregarded, but now Suzanne's method of eating is accepted as a standard and sensible way to gain control over your weight and guide you on the path to lifelong health. A healthy diet is vital, today more than ever before. In fact, more positive application of our desire to reduce the incidence of cancers should be directed toward diet. According to the American Cancer Society, more than 50 percent of cancers in the United States are linked to obesity, including breast cancer and colon cancer.

I admire the message that Suzanne gives in *The Sexy Years*. Hor-mone therapy, the natural bioidentical way, does require a bit more effort. But rather than being overwhelming, it's an effort that's well spent. The fact that she has shared her personal experiences with people on a variety of subjects has probably helped far more people than she will ever know. It is a beautiful way to use her celebrity status. Suzanne speaks with a more powerful voice than many of us who have spent years in laboratories and behind office walls. She serves as a vital example of what we all can strive to achieve.

The practice of medicine is headed down a new road, one of self-directed health care, assisted by the guidance of health care educators willing to apply their communication skills. In my opinion, Suzanne Somers has earned that distinction. It's becoming more important for patients to take an active role and form alliances with their providers. As a doctor, I know it is more important to make patients comfortable with the information we can provide them than to intimidate them into following our instructions. The average person must be able to individualize his or her health care requests according to personal needs and beliefs. They're doing it anyway by self-adjustment of doses, refusal to refill prescriptions, or simply discontinuation of treatment. We have the obligation to rebuild their confidence by providing knowledge and fostering communication. Menopause and andropause are life-changing events in the lives of women and men. They are the least understood medical mystery but one of paramount importance because we're all living longer now than ever before. I am committed to helping women understand their choices and guiding them through the decision-making process.

Suzanne Somers is committed to helping women and men, and this book is on point in approaching the second half of life with joy and anticipation. The inherent bliss of perfectly balanced hormones is available to all who desire it. This passage requires work and careful consideration on the part of the doctor and patient, but together each individual can find his or her exquisite quality of life. The second half of life can indeed be the best ever, if hormone balance is truly understood. My enthusiasm for this message is unwavering.

THE
sexy
years

INTRODUCTION

I love being a grown-up, yet as a woman I have been programmed to dread this passage of life—the middle years, when I would become an over-the-hill, dried-up, bitchy, menopausal, sexless, useless, discarded, once-attractive, no-longer-desirable, stringy-haired, wrinkly old lady. That's what society tells us we will become. No wonder we women have been on a constant search for that secret elixir, anything promising the fountain of youth, whether it be the newest creams, potions, plastic surgery, or dream product that will give us just a few more years before the sentence of invisibility becomes our destiny. Make no mistake: Growing up is not for sissies. Doing it well takes work. As with any worthwhile endeavor, the time we put into preparing for growth and change determines the outcome. Medicine is changing so rapidly that as individuals we must be proactive about our health in order to take advantage of the newest breakthroughs. We're not supposed to feel worn out; we're not predisposed to get the diseases associated with aging. We are supposed to be happy and healthy, and if we work at it, there's no reason we shouldn't be.

All my life I have prided myself on being a person who looks at life with a positive spin. I have refused to be a victim, whether faced with an alcoholic father, a teenage pregnancy and subsequent divorce from the father, the struggles of single motherhood with no consistent job, a tangled affair with a married man, a catapult into stardom only to be cut short by a scandalous contract negotiation, a fight to regain my career, dealing with the complexities of blending two families into one, even a battle with a life-threatening disease. Through it all I have searched for the lessons that life brings. My abusive father unwittingly taught me to fight and believe in myself, even when I felt no one else did. My son has been my greatest gift, and I believe he was sent to me to keep me alive through one of the most difficult periods in my life. An affair turned into my future husband, my lifelong partner and ultimate soul mate. The years I lived as a destitute mother have kept me grateful for all the blessings I now have in my life. When *Three's Company* ended, I was forced to look deep within myself and develop other areas of my career beyond being a television actress—as a stage actress, an author, a lecturer, and ultimately a brand name. The hard years of blending stepchildren have paid off, as we now have a unified family that is my greatest joy . . . with six grandchildren! And cancer taught me about the enormous love that surrounds me, that I can overcome any obstacle, and to enjoy the sweet moments of each and every day.

I wasn't looking for another lesson in life, but you never know when they will arrive. Here I was, merrily handling the aging process and being grateful for the wisdom I gained in exchange for the crow's-feet around my eyes. The children were grown with families of their own, and I had decided this was going to be the best phase of my life yet. I would grow old gracefully and teach those around me that we don't have to dread this time of life. Then, suddenly, the Seven Dwarfs of Menopause arrived at my door without warning: Itchy, Bitchy, Sweaty, Sleepy, Bloated, Forgetful, and All-Dried-Up. One by one they crept into my own private cottage in the woods and started to take over my life. For me, the first to arrive was Itchy. I developed this itch on my right calf that was so irritating, I wanted to scratch the skin right off my body. Then Bitchy came to my door. No longer was my PMS contained to one or two days a month—it felt like constant PMS. Then I would swing from Bitchy to weepy—for God's sake, what was wrong with me? *Ding-dong* . . . It's the middle of the night, and Sweaty has crawled into bed with me. Oh, yes, Sweaty brought embarrassing hot flashes and introduced me to night sweats where it seemed as if a faucet had been attached between my breasts. Of course Sweaty brought about Sleepy because I was tired all the time. I would wake up so many times in the night and not be able to get back to sleep. Bloated crept in slowly. My once-svelte figure got thick through the middle section, even though I was following my weight-loss program that had worked so well for so many years! I can't quite remember when Forgetful arrived, but one day my brain stopped working. I considered myself a pretty focused woman until Forgetful came and I could not keep a coherent thought in my brain. I remember doing an interview, and I couldn't remember a single question to ask! Am I getting Alzheimer's? I wondered. Last, All-Dried-Up slowly encroached upon my happy marriage. This was probably the most unpleasant of the dwarf family. Sex was no longer on the top of my list . . . or on my list at all. My husband would give me that knowing look, and I would think, "Frankly, I'd rather have a smoothie."

Yes, menopause had hit me like a ton of bricks, and I was completely unprepared. My mother certainly never talked about it. I had no training for this! Our mates are just as unprepared. At first our men may be sympathetic, but they quickly tire of the complaining, worn-out rag of a woman formerly known as the love of their life. To alleviate our symptoms, we seek answers from our doctors and get conflicting reports about hormone replacement therapy. Yes, it will take away the symptoms, but what are the risks? I don't want cancer, but I'm so depressed! Most conventional wisdom in our fix-the-symptom medical community leads women to synthetic hormones in combination with Prozac or Paxil (which is simply Prozac turned into a pink pill for women with PMD or menopausal symptoms) to help them through this passage. This is not a cure, by any means.

So why, you ask, would I call this book *The Sexy Years*? Doesn't sound so sexy yet, eh? Because I have found the elixir—the juice of youth that has sent the Seven Dwarfs of Menopause off to the coal mines never to return! I handled this crisis like every other one in my life. I was not going to let it beat me. I would not go silently into the night and let go of the woman I wanted to be for myself and for my husband. So I fought for an answer that would work for me. I dug into research on the subject and talked to as many doctors as I could. One thing I have learned is that medicine is not black and white. No one doctor has the right answer for everyone: You must gather all the information and make the decision you feel is best for you. There are hundreds of ways to make brownies . . . you must find the recipe that you think tastes the best.

Personally, I have found my answer. What was it that sent those wretched dwarfs packing? Natural bioidentical hormones. As you will read in the coming chapters, I have learned that natural bioidentical hormones are the secret to handling this passage of life (not the synthetic hormones that only slap a Band-Aid on your menopausal symptoms and have garnered so much controversy in medical studies, and certainly not black cohosh and yams). Once I got my hormones balanced by actually replacing the lost hormones, I lost Itchy. My mood leveled off and I lost Bitchy. I got control of my body temperature and Sweaty went away. With balanced hormones Sleepy disappeared and I recovered the glorious ability to sleep through the night. Day by day my body slimmed down, so I could say good-bye to Bloated. I regained my sharp thinking—farewell, Forgetful. And the look in my husband's eye was returned with a wink and lovingly reciprocated, as I happily banished All-Dried-Up.

I am a testament that it is possible to take on this passage of life and embrace it. I will tell you that you do not have to take this transition lying down. You have choices! You have options! You have solutions! In this book I share with you my journey and several stories of what other women are dealing with so that you may find your own answers. I have interviewed cutting-edge doctors who have provided further information that natural bioidentical hormones are the way to go. This book gives you a battle plan to conquer this beast and come out the other side with a victorious song of praise.

It takes commitment to approach this time of life with grace, anticipation, and a willingness to really look at the truth about yourself, not only physically but on an emotional level as well. The amount of work you are willing to put into this passage will determine your happiness quotient—but wouldn't all the work be worth it if, in the end, you knew your life would be the best it had ever been? I can't speak for any age group but my own; however, I do know each passage brings its rewards if you know what it is you want from your life. If you grieve for your once-perfect body and your twenty-year-old looks, this book will not help you. But if what you desire is confidence, extraordinary good health, happiness, peace, serenity, fulfillment, great looks, a fabulous body, lots of fun, and a sex life like you've never had before, then by all means read on.

There is only one thing you need to know before you start reading, and it is that it's up to you. No one can help you into the next passage except you, and that is the challenge and the fun. What you resist persists; what you fear is what you draw to you. If you fear growing up, if you are afraid of evolving, you are doomed to be an immature adult. There is nothing more unattractive than an immature adult. These are the people whose lives have gone off track because they are foolishly chasing their youth instead of accepting change. But life is a flow, and we must follow it wherever it leads us. The happiest people are those who can put this into a positive perspective. Everything you think you have lost is really your opportunity to gain. It's looking at the glass as half full instead of half empty.

There is no need to dread menopause. The work I have done to understand this time of my life has brought me to a place of absolute joy. I am balanced and on track, and—no kidding—this passage has become the most glorious time of my life.

As you read this book, you will see that, across the board, it is the women of menopausal age on natural bioidentical hormones who are enjoying the greatest health and quality of life. When you get your hormones balanced and actually replace the hormones you have lost in the aging process, you will experience the bliss, vitality, sexual vigor, and excitement that I have come to experience at this age. There is no reason to suffer through this hormonal passage, and so many women are suffering. Menopause is a challenge and it takes a lot of work to manage, but once you understand how to balance your hormones, it becomes simple. You'll wonder why you did not approach menopause this way in the first place. Honest to God! This period of my life, menopause and all, is the best I have ever felt.

Come with me on this exciting journey. I want to share everything I have learned in my search for answers. This is exciting information that you can then pass on to your daughters, sisters, and women in general. And let's not forget the men in our lives. Wait until you learn about male menopause, andropause. It's a very real passage that is highly misunderstood. In this book I will explain not only women's hormonal needs, but also men's needs for the sex hormones testosterone, estrogen (yes, estrogen), progesterone, and DHEA; and this information is life-changing. We men and women are in this together, so let's help one another.

There is so much misinformation and ignorance about this time in our lives. As baby boomers we have always demanded a better quality of life. After all, we are the generation who burned our bras; we demanded equality in the workplace; we are the first generation of women who wanted to understand the complexities of our feelings and used therapy as a learning tool. So now we've reached a time in our lives when women of prior generations suffered in silence. That silence has led to ignorance and confusion about menopause. But why shouldn't we demand optimal treatments and the best information available about this transition? Let's get it on the table. Let's let go of the shame. Let's make this the best time. Let's be creative about how we present ourselves at this age. Let's look at life as though the glass is half full. Then we can truthfully pass on to the next generation (by our example) the message that this is an enviable passage.

Imagine that you can enjoy your sexuality today in a way that will make those early years of intensity, new love, and overwhelming magic seem like child's play. You know why? Because it *was* child's play! At my present age the fears, the guilt, the embarrassment, and the worry no longer factor into my sexuality, because my life is on track emotionally and hormonally. I'm feeling frisky, and I want to tell you how and why. As I said, growing up is not for sissies. Achieving this bliss will require an honest look into the part you are playing in the drama of your life. It will require you to take an honest look at how you are managing your health. Once you get your hormones in balance, we will look to see what behavioral patterns you have created that are preventing you from becoming your happiest self, a process that requires absolute truthfulness to your self about yourself. What is it about you that you would prefer no one ever know? This is a good place to start. This is where healing can begin. These are the steps toward enjoying *the sexy years*.

PART I

THE hormone connection

1

CANCER

The last words I ever thought I'd hear about myself were "You have breast cancer." It was as though someone had dropped a load of lead on my head. I felt stunned. This is something that happens to other people, I thought. Not me. I figured, I am healthy, I eat right, I have exercised all my life. My sister being diagnosed with breast cancer four years earlier was just a fluke. I mean, other than her, there is no history of breast cancer in my family, I reasoned. How could this be happening?

Every year since I turned forty I have been going to the USC/ Norris Comprehensive Cancer Center and Hospital in Los Angeles. I always looked forward to seeing my doctor, Mel Silverstein, who created the concept of the breast centers in this country. He is a nice guy and has committed his life to the care of women's breasts. My husband always jokingly tells him he is the luckiest guy around because he spends his days feeling women's bosoms.

It was time for my yearly mammogram, and I had been religious about having annual checkups since I turned forty. Because I had been so diligent, I cockily assumed that I was immune to the disease. After all, keeping such a vigilant check on my breasts would ensure that even if there was a problem, we would find it before it ever had a chance to take hold. The nurse pulled and squeezed, flattened, and pressed my poor aching breasts into positions no breast was meant to endure. But it was for a good cause, and all women know that the discomfort and humiliation are worth it in the long run, because this examination is about life, health, and prevention.

"Well, I don't see anything to worry about," Dr. Silverstein announced cheerily after looking at my mammogram.

I felt relieved, even though I hadn't even considered the possibility. Now I could go on with my life for another year knowing I had beaten the statistics once again.

I went into the changing room and hurriedly put my clothes back on. I had a busy day ahead of me—meetings with the various vendors for my jewelry business, the skin care line, updates on the fitness business, costume fittings, and a band rehearsal to get ready for an upcoming date in Las Vegas the following week. I was filled with energy and vitality.

"Suzanne?" I heard Dr. Silverstein call through the changing room door.

"Yes," I answered.

"You know, you've got such cystic breasts—lumps and bumps everywhere. How about having an ultrasound for good measure?"

I opened the door, wondering why this would be necessary. "Wasn't everything okay with my mammography?" I asked.

"Sure," Dr. Silverstein said good-naturedly. "It's just that we have this new state-of-the-art ultrasound machine. I just paid half a million dollars for it; and what the heck, let's take a look for good measure."

Why not, I reasoned. I was there, and it would only take another half hour. Surely I could fit this into my busy schedule. My health was more important than anything.

I lay down on a stationary bed in the ultrasound room, feeling no alarm, since this was just for "good measure." The technician rubbed on some cold, gooey liquid (a conductive fluid) and then began a gentle movement on my breasts with a wand about the size of a curling iron. She kept rubbing back and forth for some time in one particular area on my upper right breast. Then she excused herself and said she would be back in a couple of moments. I still felt no alarm. I had been through these exams before. Often we found cysts that were filled with fluid, which were then drained with a needle. Not the most pleasant experience, but part of the routine. I wasn't worried. Even when the technician returned with the radiologist to further probe my now rather sore and over-worked breast, I heard myself telling them, "Not to worry. I always have these cysts; they're just filled with fluid."

The tone in the room turned noticeably serious, and I was at a loss as to why everyone seemed so intense.

"We see something here we don't like, so we're going to stick a needle into it to see what we come up with."

Frankly, I felt relieved. It's the same old thing, I thought. "I've had needles before," I told her cheerfully.

"Well, this is going to be a bit more uncomfortable than what you are used to. We are using a bigger needle, and I will try my best not to hurt you."

The doctor inserted the needle, and this was indeed different. It felt like a carving knife being plunged into my flesh.

"Yeow!" I said, trying to stifle the fact that this hurt like hell.

"You're going to feel a little pop, like a cap gun going off inside of you," she told me. "This way we can gather a piece of tissue for biopsy. Okay, ready?" she asked.

Pop! Wow! It hurt . . . a lot! It felt more like a real gun going off in my breast. Then I felt the needle ripping through my breast while the doctor pulled with all her strength to get the needle out.

"Oh, my God!" I blurted out. "That is painful."

"I know; I'm sorry," she said. "Unfortunately, we are going to have to do this several more times."

Several insertions later we were finished.

The pain was unbelievable. My breasts felt like punching bags. Okay, at least now we've done it, and I can get on with my day, I thought. As I dressed, I decided to tell Dr. Silverstein that he should have prepared me for the pain a little better. In fact, after all the pulling and probing, I wasn't feeling very cheery; and in thinking about it, I felt a little angry that Dr. Silverstein had downplayed the hurt quotient. Carefully I pulled on my jacket, which was no easy feat because of the pain in my breast, and then opened the door of the changing room. Standing in the hallway just outside were Dr. Silverstein, the radiologist, and the nurse, all with serious looks on their faces.

Dr. Silverstein took my hand sensitively and said, "We hope you will be okay."

"What?" I asked, bewildered.

"It doesn't look good," Dr. Silverstein said.

"What do you mean?" I asked. I could feel my heart pounding.

"Of course, we're waiting for the pathology report to come back in a few hours," Dr. Silverstein explained, "but from what I can see, I think we should make plans for surgery."

I experienced the next hours as though I were under water. I heard and saw everything, but it was filtered, distant. I was in shock. So many decisions had to be made. They had found a malignant tumor, 2.4 centimeters in size. It was lodged deep in my chest and had not been detected. The doctors thought it had been growing for approximately ten years. How could the mammogram have missed something so large? I kept asking myself.

Cancer is lonely. The decisions to be made are too serious and too monumental to be passed on to anyone. These were decisions I had to make. It was unfair of me even to ask Alan, my husband, what he thought I should do. Luckily, we had caught it soon enough so it didn't look as though they would have to perform a mastectomy. They would remove the tumor and some lymph nodes from under my arm. If the margins were clean, they would not have to remove the breast. I never thought that I would have my own cancer doctor; but now I had an oncologist, Dr. Waisman. I liked him. He was wise, sensitive, and smart.

I was still in a daze. Only this morning I had been getting ready to go to Las Vegas in a week with my show, and now it all seemed insignificant and unimportant. Alan and I sat in the waiting room, not knowing how to feel. I kept thinking, One day life is perfect; the next day it's as if all the balls have been thrown into the air, and you have no idea where they will land. I'd never given dying any thought. It's what happens somewhere down the line a long time from now. For the first time in my life, I was faced with the possibility of my own mortality.

We drove home in a stunned silence. Alan and I walked on the beach for a long time. Our arms were wrapped around each other, giving support. We were in this together. I couldn't think. I was being asked by so many what I wanted to do, but I couldn't give them any answers. I didn't know.

The following morning I awakened from what seemed to be a nightmare, and suddenly I knew I had to take charge. It was my body, and I *wanted* to be in charge. I called my endocrinologist and dear friend, Dr. Diana Schwarzbein, to fill her in on my condition. This was war. I began a visualization of my tumor. Inside the tumor I saw this cowardly, creepy person hiding. Every time I saw him even try to step out of the encapsulated tumor, I would yell in my mind with all the venom I could muster, *Don't even try to leave this tumor, or I'll fucking kill you.* Then I visualized the cowardly little cancer cells shrink with fear and step back inside the tumor. I know it sounds weird, but at that moment I didn't know how to keep the cancer at bay, and this was the only way I could feel that I had any control over it.

Next, I started making phone calls. My agent, Al Lowman, said, "You should talk to Selma Schimmel."

"Who's that?" I asked.

"She's one of my authors who has written a lot about breast cancer."

Selma told me about Dr. Avrum Bluming, who was doing research with women and breast cancer and hormone replacement therapy (HRT), albeit with synthetic hormones. I did not want to give up my hormones. As you will find out in the next few chapters I have expended a great deal of effort getting my chemicals balanced and learning about natural hormones; now, upon diagnosis, I was being told that hormones had to be stopped because of my breast cancer. I knew what that meant relative to the quality of my life, and I was not about to go back to feeling the way I had before I got my hormones balanced.

I started to gather doctors. Dr. Waisman came highly recommended, but I wanted other opinions. I told Dr. Waisman about Dr. Bluming, and he said that not only did he know him, but he was working with him on a study of the connection between women with breast cancer and hormone replacement therapy. Okay, this is good, I thought.

I was on the phone constantly. Cancer is like a job. The treatments are inexact. There is the "common course" of treatment, but so far everything I was being told about the common course was not appealing to me. I knew of too many people who were on the chemotherapy merry-go-round. Chemo seems to make people in treatment more ill; and frankly, it scared me to death. I was afraid of what it would do to the good cells; and I can't say that I wasn't more than a little afraid of the harshness of the treatment. First there's the hair loss and then the sickly color the complexion takes on; then there's the damage done to the parts of the body that until this time were functioning properly. The idea of ingesting potent chemicals was abhorrent and frightening to me. I am against putting chemicals into the body unless absolutely necessary, and I wanted to be sure that this was the only option before I took on something so radical.

Then it was suggested that after surgery I would take the drug tamoxifen for the next five years as a preventative. The only problem I found in doing my research was that this drug would probably make me depressed for much of the duration, plus there was a 40 percent increased risk of heart attack, stroke, and pulmonary embolism. All this for only a 10 percent greater chance that the cancer would not recur? Didn't sound like very good odds to me. I felt weary. So much information to gather, so much authority to weigh. It would be easier to just sit back and let all of "them" handle it for me. That is what I would have done in my younger years. I would have assumed that they knew better. I would have followed the common course. But things were different now. I was a grown-up, and the privilege that comes with having lived this long is the realization that no one knows better than I what I want to do with my body. I have worked too hard all my life to undo the damage of my childhood, to get out from under the grip of having been raised by an abusive alcoholic, to make something of my life, to raise a child on my own, to endure the pain of blending families, to see my career knocked out from under me in a war of egos, only to come out the loser in the whole deal. I could not have known that those earlier ordeals would give me the strength to fight this giant war now raging inside my body.

The big revelation that comes with maturity is that life is a series of highs and lows, and it's during the low points of life that you have breakthroughs. Through the negatives we are given the opportunities to have that "aha" moment where we figure out what we don't want in our lives. I didn't want to live my life as a victim; I didn't want to use the excuse that I coulda or shoulda or woulda had a great life, but I had some bad luck. It has always been the "bad luck" or the negatives in my life that have taught me and shaped me, and I wasn't going to lose this time around. Cancer was going to be my blessing. I was going to learn and grow and *survive* my way.

Surgery, frankly, is the easy part. I knew I needed to get this tumor out of me. I wanted that, and so did my doctors. It's a painful surgery because a lot of the prep is done while you are awake without the benefit of painkillers—like the wires they insert in and around your breast to create a sort of "cradle" for the tumor so the surgeon knows the exact perimeters of the diseased area.

When you have breast cancer, they know up front that it is malignant, confirmed through the biopsy and subsequent pathology. What you don't know is how far it's gone. If cancer cells are found in the lymph nodes, your chances of survival decrease. Because of this, there's definitely a lot of anxiety surrounding the surgery. I couldn't get over the déjà vu aspect of these happenings. One of the poems I wrote for my first book of poetry, *Touch Me,* in 1973, was called "For the Moment." It had to do with enjoying the moment, for you never know what tomorrow might bring.

My diagnosis and the way it had suddenly consumed my life had happened in a matter of days. Just last weekend I was fine and strong and healthy, and today I was being wheeled into unknown territory, having no idea of the outcome. I was doing my best. So far I had refused to give up my natural bioidentical hormones. As a result of intense research, it is my belief that it is an environment of balanced hormones that prevents disease, so why would I want to give up the very thing that could help me win this war? My surgeon and cancer doctors were distressed over my decision. None of them had ever known of anyone who had done this. But belief is a potent motivator. I envisioned the hormones standing like sentries, shoulder to shoulder, forming a protective circle around each of my precious organs. To me they were the front line. I needed their help. That was my first tactic. The other decisions regarding chemotherapy, radiation, and the follow-up drugs would be made when I was post-op and had more time to gather my thoughts. But first I had to get the cancer out of me.

I remember the cocktail. Oh my, the drug they give you to put you out for surgery is a real thrill. I had Valium and then Demerol. Once that stuff hits your veins, you haven't a care in the world. As I drifted off into space, I can recall the worried faces of my husband, Alan, and my stepdaughter, Leslie, standing over me, their hands holding mine. I told them I loved them, and the next thing I knew it was three hours later and someone handed me a telephone receiver. It was Barry Manilow.

"Are you okay?" he asked, clearly concerned.

"You were so wonderful on your special last night," I told him. "I loved how you sang the closing song a cappella. It was so courageous and moving."

"I can't believe you," he said, stunned. "You're just being wheeled out of surgery, and you're telling me about my television special."

I started mumbling incoherently, and Barry said, "Let me talk to Alan so I can find out how you are."

That's when I heard Alan telling Barry that they felt they got it all and there was no cancer in the lymph nodes. In my drugged state I could feel the tension leave my body, and I fell into a deep, peaceful sleep until the next day.

My children took care of me. My daughter-in-law, Caroline, made delicious turkey soup for my recovery. This was the worst possible disease I could have gotten for Caroline. She lost her mother to breast cancer when she was a little girl, then her stepmother to ovarian cancer; and then her surrogate mother, her aunt, died of breast cancer. I have always assured her that I would be with her for her entire life, that I was her designated earth mother and would always be there for her. Even with my diagnosis I knew I was going to keep that promise.

My grandchildren filled my large king-size bed with their giggles; yet somehow they knew something was up. Camelia, my four-year-old, whispered into my ear, "I'm sorry you have an oowie on your booby, Zannie." They all wanted to see what it looked like.

Alan stayed in bed with me the whole time I was recovering. He's like that. He brought soup and damp, cool towels and woke me when it was time for my medication.

Bruce, my son, was traumatized. I kept reassuring him I was going to be okay. We had been through so much together in our lives, and the idea of his mother being sick was hard for him to handle.

My stepson, Stephen, and his wife, Olivia, came with the children. I felt so blessed. After all the work of bringing the two families together, Alan's children from his first marriage and my son, Bruce, I knew at this moment that we had succeeded. I could see it in their faces. This was the first blessing of cancer.

Now the decisions had to be made. Two of my doctors wanted me to start chemotherapy. Dr. Waisman felt that surgery, radiation, follow-up drugs, and discontinuing hormones would be sufficient. I had found the tumor early. I now realize that is the difference between living and dying. If this tumor had been allowed to grow inside of me for another year until my next mammogram, I would most certainly have had to undergo a mastectomy and harsh chemotherapy. Because of early detection, my margins were clean;

in other words, the surgeon found no evidence that the cancer had spread. This was the best-case scenario of a bad situation. The bad news was that my type of cancer had a high return rate. What I chose as aftercare was extremely important. I was struck over and over by the fact that my wonderful breast surgeon, Dr. Silverstein, had saved my life by encouraging me to have an additional check on the ultrasound. This is the beauty of living in a highly advanced technological age. Technology is about thinking progressively, always moving forward. This was significant to me, because as I began to gather information, I was leaning more toward thinking my preventative choices were going to differ from those of my doctors in some areas.

One week after surgery, I had my first post-operative exam. Both my doctors were pleased with the healing of the wound. It was the first time I had actually seen what had been done. Dr. Silverstein was able to save my breast by filling the huge gap that had been created when removing such a large tumor with the fat from the underside of my breast. Even though this breast was now slightly smaller than the other one, my doctor had done an excellent job of making it look beautiful. It was full and shaped well, and the scar was stitched to perfection.

"We have to talk about your options," Dr. Silverstein said. "We've gone over it with you, and we feel that chemotherapy would ensure your recovery; and radiation is a must. Also, you have to stop taking your hormones and start taking daily doses of tamoxifen."

"As you can imagine," I told them, "I have done nothing but think about this all week. I've spoken to my other two doctors and gathered information from them. These are big decisions, and I know time is of the essence; but I can't jump into treatment until I feel I've explored all the avenues. At the moment, I don't want to take chemotherapy—I'm afraid of what it will do to my *good* cells—and this aftercare drug you've recommended sounds terrible to me. I mean, is this the best they have to offer women? The next five years are important ones to me. I'm still young, and I want to enjoy what's left of my youth. I don't want to feel depressed and nauseated all the time. I want my hair. I don't want to be or look sick. These treatments will affect the quality of my life without a promise of success, and it most certainly will affect my ability to work."

The doctors were kind, sensitive, and respectful. We talked for a long, long time. "It's all up to you, Suzanne," Dr. Waisman said. "We will work with you and support you with whatever treatment you choose."

Now all I had to do was decide.

I must have called Dr. Diana Schwarzbein every couple of hours over the next few weeks. She helped me with research on every option. She sent me the latest studies, just as she had been doing for the last several years for my Somersize weight loss program. Giving up hormones was the biggest decision.

"I don't want to stop taking them," I told Diana over and over.

I talked to another doctor and told him the same thing. He said, "I have to recommend that you stop taking hormones, and I have to recommend that you take chemotherapy, radiation, and tamoxifen. There is a new drug called Herceptin, but it's not right for your kind of cancer." Then he leaned in to me and said, "I *have* to recommend that you do these things."

I looked at him for a while, thinking, and then asked, "Are you telling me to read between the lines?" The look on his face said yes.

I suddenly realized what he was saying. Legally, because we live in such a litigious society, he had to recommend the "common course." But he was trying to tell me to follow my instincts.

"Tell me something," I said. "If I were in my thirties and my body was making a full complement of hormones and I had this same cancer, would you remove my ovaries?"

"Of course not," he replied.

"Then why would you ask me to stop taking my natural bioidentical hormones, which are replacing the ones I have lost in the aging process?" I asked.

He paused a long time and then said thoughtfully, "We don't know."

The air between us was still for a moment. It was true: there were no studies to tell doctors in this country anything to the contrary, and I realized my doctor was being responsible. But in pursuing the logic of my thoughts, I realized he was also giving me precious information.

"Thank you," I said gratefully. I had my answer. Women are deprived of their hormones when they have cancer because it is thought to be safer, legally, to take them off hormones *in case* hormones feed tumors. Also, I knew most doctors thought of "hormones" as the synthetic type, which are really not hormones at all. Synthetic "hormones" create hormonal imbalance (which I will explain later in the book), and hormonal imbalance leaves you open to disease. I was taking natural hormones, and my system was in balance. Now I was on to something.

I called Diana Schwarzbein. "Isn't it an environment of balanced hormones that prevents disease?"

"Absolutely," she said, and went on to explain. That's why young people do not get the diseases of aging, because aging is loss of hormones. It's like watering a plant. With water the plant flourishes if it is in the right environment for itself. If you stop watering the plant, it will continue to grow; but over time it will stop looking so good, and eventually the plant will keel over and die. The same thing happens to humans. As we lose our hormones in the aging process, we continue to look and feel good, much like the plant; but eventually, without our hormones, which provide nourishment to our organs, we start to have problems. A disease here, a medical problem there; and eventually we die because we are no longer being nurtured, nourished, and fertilized by our hormones. It is then that our bodies give out on us.

In my youth I would have followed the doctor's orders. As a grown-up I had the abilities to gather information and decipher. And now I knew what I wanted to do.

I called Diana. "I've made my decision," I told her. "I'm going to continue to take my hormones, I am not going to take chemotherapy, I *am* going to have six weeks of radiation, and I am not going to take tamoxifen."

She paused for a while and then said, "You know, I've tried to walk in your shoes for the last few weeks; and although I would not and could not tell you what to do, I thought about what I would do in your situation. I know I would absolutely be making the same decisions as you. I believe your thinking is not only on track, but cutting-edge."

I cannot tell you the relief I felt at hearing her say that. I was dealing with my life, a life that I have worked hard at correcting and fixing so that I could be my best and healthiest self. I didn't want to blow it. I didn't want to make decisions about my life that could possibly shorten it or harm me. Diana is one of the people I admire and respect deeply. I knew she would not say anything to me that she did not mean. Now I felt secure in the treatment schedule I had prescribed for myself.

I'm out of estrogen and I have a gun.

2

HORMONES

Getting cancer reinforced the importance of being proactive about my health. I knew I needed to work extra hard to keep my body in balance as I aged by continuing my regimen of natural bioidentical hormones. I became very involved in learning about hormones when I started to experience the symptoms of menopause a few years ago. If you're in or approaching middle age, you know exactly what I'm talking about. Our skin begins to change (enter Itchy); we lose vaginal lubrication (here comes All-Dried-Up); we start getting aches and pains that don't go away; we are hot, then cold (Sweaty is really fun); and we can't sleep, which puts us in an unbearable mood over time because we are exhausted. In addition, as we lose our hormones in the aging process, we leave ourselves open to a variety of diseases of aging, and then the Big Unmentionable—many of us lose our sex drive.

Menopause (or, as I call it, men-on-pause) is traumatic. I always wondered why men leave their wives of long standing at middle age. It's not because their wives are getting older or that they don't look good anymore; they leave because women become impossible to live with during this passage. Plus, a lot of women have *no* interest in sex. I experienced this phenomenon. Honestly, it was like losing an old friend. I felt a sadness and a sense of betrayal, because women of prior generations never prepared me for this loss. Why hasn't this been discussed? I wondered. Am I the only woman to ever have this experience? I think this subject has been in the closet so long that women have chosen to endure it silently. It's like admitting that the reason Bitchy is here today is that you have PMS. No one likes to admit that because it connotes weakness, that we are out of control. And pity the poor man who suggests that you might be unreasonable today because of your period. This could be construed as grounds for war.

For over thirty years, the sexual part of the relationship between my husband and me has always been thrilling. It has been where we connect intimately, where we have experienced an indescribable closeness, trust, passion, and sexual adventure. It has been where we solve our problems; where we allow each other to be exactly what we are feeling at that particular moment. Suddenly, in our thirty-first year together, with no warning, I felt dead inside. I didn't understand it. Where I once was always in the mood, now I felt nothing. I did it, but I felt nothing. My friskiness was gone, my sense of adventure left me. I had no energy. I felt like crying all the time. I didn't want to get out of bed in the morning. I couldn't remember anything. I was afraid I had early-onset Alzheimer's disease because I couldn't hold a thought. Itchy appeared and my skin itched horribly and I found it impossible to sleep for more than fifteen minutes at a time; and then Sweaty appeared and I would awaken soaking wet from hot flashes. What a life, huh? What had happened?

I didn't completely understand at the time, but what was happening to me is common to most women as we get older. I had zeroed out hormonally. I was no longer making my full complement of hormones. Because of that, I had no life-restoring nutrients feeding me metabolically. My organs were shutting down from lack of nutrients. These are strictly lay terms; but for you and me, it's easier to understand with this terminology. We are our hormones. Without them we die. In fact, aging is the loss of hormones. From the middle to late thirties (and it differs by a few years from person to person), we make a full complement of hormones. Then we hit perimenopause, and our hormones begin to fluctuate as they start to diminish, until they get close to zeroing out in menopause.

Women lose 90 percent of their hormones over a two-year period, once we begin to go into menopause. No wonder we feel crazy!

This is a difficult passage of life. All the balance of your life gets jumbled. Suddenly your husband doesn't understand you anymore. He says things like "What's wrong with you?" Your insides are screaming, *I don't know, I don't know.* On top of it, here comes the weight gain; every day your favorite pants are getting tighter and tighter. You feel dumpy and you start to notice what great shape all the other women are in. You remember when you looked like that. What has changed? You are eating the same as before, maybe even less. You've stopped with the desserts; you're trying to exercise, but you're so tired from not sleeping; and the hot flashes—those embarrassing hot flashes—wake you up continuously all through the night. You feel ugly and fat, and now you have no desire for sex. Is it because you are so tired? That's what you keep telling him, because he's starting to get irritated that "you're never in the mood anymore." Secretly you're wondering also, *Why* don't I want to have sex? You do it because you don't want him to be angry with you all the time, but you can't *feel* anything. *Nothing!* All there is is a sensation that something is inside you, but it might as well be the probe the gynecologist inserts, because the sensation is about the same; and it isn't a sexual feeling.

I felt this. I was *dead* inside. It was sad and lonely, humiliating, confusing, and isolating. I didn't want to talk to my husband about it because I was afraid he would find the whole thing such a turnoff.

I remember Howard Stern asking me on his radio show one morning, "Are you in menopause?" He asked in such a way that he made it sound disgusting. I felt the shame women talk about regarding the subject. I answered, sounding equally disgusted, "Of course not," hoping my astonishment at the question would ward off his suspicions. Howard was not unique. Most men find menopause icky. If they are with us during this passage, it reminds them that they, along with us, are aging; and if they are young, like

Howard, they know only what they have heard—that women turn into lunatics during this passage and it's best to avoid them at all costs. Several times in my life I have heard men referring to an older woman as a "dried-up old menopausal bitch." So we're supposed to be looking forward to this passage?

Why must we do penance for coming to this age? It seems unfair to me that the payoff for a woman who has spent much of her life happily devoted to raising her children and being a good wife is to turn into such a monumental bitch that no one in the family wants to have anything to do with her. What kind of payoff is that?

In the research for my first Somersize book, *Eat Great, Lose Weight,* I knew the key to understanding weight loss was an understanding of the hormone insulin. I also knew that if one hormone in the system is off, then the entire system is out of whack. I knew that hormones were behind the symptoms that I and all other women experience when we hit middle age, but it was clear to me, from watching what was happening to women I knew and from my research, that for the most part the medical community didn't have a clue how to deal with hormones and menopause.

The most logical source of information for women about their health is their gynecologist. Unfortunately, few gynecologists are versed in natural bioidentical hormone replacement. In fact, if they haven't specialized, they don't know much about the hormonal system at all. Most gynecologists and doctors other than endocrinologists who have chosen to specialize in the hormonal system, have had four hours of study devoted to learning about this crucial internal system. So many gynecologists go with the accepted program—they find that once a woman is put on a synthetic pharmaceutical (drug) hormone, like Prempro (the combination of Premarin and Provera), or Premarin alone, she stops complaining about the uncomfortable symptoms. If she continues to complain, Prozac, Paxil, or some other form of antidepressant is prescribed. Again, she stops complaining and lives in a lethargic, medicated state that sometimes continues for the rest of her life. The tragedy of this lack of understanding is that women taking synthetic hormones are not *replacing* lost hormones. Women are simply suppressing their symptoms while their bodies are breaking down internally from a lack of nutrients being supplied to organs.

I just didn't want to take the standard course of action of synthetic hormone replacement therapy for my menopause, and I went from doctor to doctor to try to come up with a plan that would work for me. "Well, it's just a lot of guessing," my first gynecologist said. "Let's try putting you on black cohosh [a useless herb in my opinion, relative to menopause] because you don't want the synthetic hormones. Frankly, though," she said, "I don't know why you don't want to take Premarin or Provera, the synthetic hormones, because they are so much easier and there's no guesswork."

"I don't want to ingest chemicals," I told her over and over. I got no relief from this doctor, so I tried another one.

"Well, look at it this way," said the next doctor; "in days of old, women didn't live much past their childbearing years, around age forty. I mean, after all, ha, ha, ha, when you stop being able to bear children, what good are you?" He was kidding, of course, but in my state, I didn't find it very humorous.

I went on to yet another doctor, one who came highly recommended. He asked, "Why do you want to take natural hormones?"

I said, "Because I want to replace the hormones I've lost in the aging process, not simply take away the symptoms."

At that, he patted me on the head and said, "The drug companies know best, dear."

I thought, You old fool. I know that wasn't very kind of me, but come on. Often doctors are influenced in various ways by the drug companies; and because of that, many of them have forgotten that the studies they read are funded by the pharmaceutical companies that actually make the drug. So of course it all sounds wonderful! All I knew was that as I looked around, most of the women who were taking synthetic hormones were getting fat. In my own research, I already knew that hormonal imbalance is the reason one gets fat. I know that insulin is the fat-storing hormone and that insulin resistance is a result of hormonal imbalance. It was all connected. I had to find a way to not only balance my hormones by eating the Somersize way, but also to replace the hormones that I had lost. Then I would be on track.

Don't think I disregard traditional Western medicine. I am the first one in line for Western medicine when it is warranted. I would not have wanted to go through my cancer without my wonderful doctors; but I believe that in today's world it is vitally important to be proactive about your health. No one can rely upon their individual doctor to have all the answers. What I object to is doctors working outside their areas of expertise. If they don't know anything about hormones, they should say so.

The statistics are clear—we're living longer than ever before. In days of old, women died around age forty, at the end of their childbearing years. Life had many hardships then and there were few medical advances, so people died much younger than they do today. But now many of us are going to live to be in our late nineties or even our hundreds. If this is so, then we have to figure out how we are going to live a quality life for the time remaining to us. If menopause as currently experienced is any indication of what is to come, it's going to be a society of some pretty unhappy women and the people who live with them.

Enter Dr. Schwarzbein! I had heard about this woman in Santa Barbara who specialized in thyroid imbalances, diabetes, and menopause. Could it be? A doctor who gets it? Probably, I thought, she's an old bag with the usual treatments for this time of life. I was not prepared for the young, vivacious, beautiful woman who greeted me at the door. Things were about to change. Finally I was sitting before someone who understood the hormonal system. Dr. Schwarzbein told me what I inherently knew but had no basis or abilities to verify.

"Because we are living longer, we have to treat the second half of life differently," she told me.

Yes! I thought. We talked for three hours and forged what has become one of my most important relationships. Over the years she has been one of my greatest teachers. As Dr. Schwarzbein explained to me, because we are living longer, it is necessary to replace the hormones that have been lost in the aging process with natural bioidentical hormones that replicate exactly the hormones we make in our own bodies; synthetic hormones remove some of the symptoms but do very little to replace those hormones that have been lost in the aging process. Dr. Schwarzbein says that real hormones—estradiol, progesterone, testosterone, and levothyroxine, which is the thyroid hormone—are identical to those found in the human body. Synthetic hormones are drugs like Premarin, which are conjugated estrogens; Provera, which is medroxyprogesterone acetate; and methyltestosterone. These are chemicals not found in the human body. Armour thyroid contains real hormones but does not contain the correct composition.

So what does this mean? Instead of a doctor prescribing for me a synthetic "one pill fits all" type of regimen, my hormones are tracked through blood tests to see exactly where my levels are; and because of this, an endocrinologist can prescribe combinations of the real bioidentical hormones to replace what has been lost. (Don't worry, I'll explain more about all of this in the next few chapters.)

This was a revelation to me, and I was ready to get with the program and have Dr. Schwarzbein replace all my lost hormones. Who wouldn't want this? But it wasn't as simple as that. I said to Dr. Schwarzbein, "If you know what I'm missing hormonally, why don't you give me an exact dosage for my levels?"

"I can't do that," she explained. "It took a long time for you to lose these hormones, and we have to replace them gradually or else you'll feel crazy. Hormones are not to be played around with. Too much is as bad as too little. We will eventually build your levels to the perfect balance for you, but it has to be done gradually."

Each of us is made up of a completely different chemical composite from the next person. What I require is going to be different from what you require, even if our blood work shows that you and I have the exact same hormonal levels. I may require more estrogen to feel good or more or less progesterone to feel good than you might. In the next chapter, I'll talk more about how you can work with your doctor to come up with a program that works just for you. Believe it or not, one of the more exciting aspects of treating hormonal decline is working in concert with your doctor. It is up to you, the patient, to know when your body is feeling at optimum or if new blood work is required to find out if your levels have changed. When hormones are imbalanced you will not be able to operate at peak performance for your age and lifestyle.

The good news was that I started to feel relief immediately. I began to sleep better, the hot flashes subsided, and slowly my sex drive returned. My thinking also got better, and the horrible itch on my legs went away. I was still battling a little weight gain; but, luckily, I had been eating on my Somersize plan for so long that my weight was being controlled through that.

"When your hormones get in full balance," my doctor explained, "the weight gain will disappear because you already have great eating habits."

When you get your hormones balanced by taking bioidentical hormones and eating right and exercising, you will achieve your ideal body composition. We don't have to be pear shaped or apple shaped in middle age, and this alone would make natural bioidentical hormones preferable. Synthetic (drug) hormones cannot offer this to a woman. Add to that other health benefits such as more youthful skin, more energy, sharper thinking, no memory loss, fewer mood swings, less depression, less anxiety, greater muscle definition, enhanced sexuality, sleeping through the night, elimination of hot flashes, and the advantages of staving off the diseases thought to automatically accompany growing older, and it is clear that this magic "cocktail," tailored just for you, is the answer.

I was beginning to see the light. It all made such sense to me. If I were a diabetic, my doctor would not prescribe the same amount of insulin for me that he did for every other patient. Every diabetic patient needs an individualized insulin "cocktail," and this is calculated through blood work to determine exactly how much insulin is needed to balance that person's glycemic index.

The same goes for menopause. Every woman is different. Hormone levels are determined by many factors. Happiness, depression, stress, and a high-stress lifestyle are all factors determining every woman's hormone levels. I have a particularly high-stress lifestyle. I always have to "go on," whether it's for a television show, my nightclub act, or a lecture, running my businesses, or getting interviewed; and all these activities are stressful and produce a level of false adrenaline. False adrenaline levels block hormone production. Therefore, at times I have to have blood work done more often to determine if during this period I need to add or take away either estradiol or progesterone. It is this constant tracking due to my high-stress lifestyle that allows me to enjoy the bliss that comes with balanced hormones. In the next few chapters I'll explain just what I mean by "constant tracking" and how I monitor my hormone levels with my doctor to stay at my peak.

It has been four years now, and I am feeling like a thirty-year-old. My hormones are perfectly balanced. I now realize that this is the secret elixir we have all been looking for. Balanced hormones are the true "fountain of youth." People are always saying to me, "You look great," and I can see them studying my face. It's simply that I have replaced the hormones I have lost, and my body, mind, and spirit are now working at optimum. It is our hormones that give us our youth, so when they are balanced, one of the positive by-products is a more youthful appearance. Since I began HRT I feel happy almost all the time. I feel a sense of balance and the serenity that comes with that. I don't feel stressed; I feel calm; I don't sweat the small stuff. I can handle a lot of things at the same time without feeling crazy because my thinking is so clear and sharp. Best of all, my sex drive is back with a vengeance. I'm in the mood for love. It's so great at this age, after thirty-five years of marriage, to look at my husband and feel all "wiggly" inside. And is he ever happy! Our kids are grown up and have started their own lives, and we have this great relationship, plus the freedom to "date" each other again just as when we first fell in love.

My life has been totally changed by taking bioidentical hormones. Do you know any woman who says synthetic hormones make them feel great? Do you know one woman on synthetic hormones who isn't complaining about her weight gain or bone loss? Doesn't it make sense to replace the hormones we are losing with exact replicas of those we make ourselves? There is no drug that can possibly be better than what we make inside our own bodies.

I hope this chapter has intrigued you. I've managed to turn my life around through HRT, and you can, too. In the next two chapters I will explain more about how hormones actually work in our bodies, what bioidentical hormones are, and how you can find the right doctor and figure out what you need to do to get with the program. This will not be an easy journey. There are very few doctors who understand real bioidentical hormone replacement. But if you are willing to do the work, the rewards will be worth it. I will walk you through my own program and give you a set of questions you can ask your own doctor. I'm not a doctor and don't pretend to be one, but I'm a passionate layperson. The next chapters will be a good introduction to the wonderful world of bioidentical HRT.

Perks of being over forty: You can live without sex, but not without glasses.

3

HOW IT WORKS

Now that you understand my passion for taking natural hormones, let's get down to business and talk about exactly what these hormones are and how they work in our bodies. Trust me, this information is fascinating and will help you better understand how your body works, so that you are able to take care of it to the best of your ability.

Let's first talk about what hormones really are and where they come from. Dr. Uzzi Reiss, a Beverly Hills gynecologist well versed in natural hormones, explained to me: "Hormones are secreted by glands, such as the adrenals, ovaries, and thyroid, that are governed by higher centers of the brain. Hormones travel throughout your bloodstream in a communication network that links the higher centers of your brain to the DNA command posts operating in the several hundred trillion cells of your adult body. On the outer and inner membranes of the cells are receptor sites that function like locks on a door. In order to get in and tell the DNA what to do, you need the right key, and hormones are the keys. They travel to specific target cells, unlock the receptor sites, and deliver their biochemical message for processing. They turn on or turn off specific cellular functions and measure cellular activity throughout the system." Clearly, hormones make things happen in the body. They are responsible for getting our cells to do the things they are supposed to do.

There are two classifications of hormones in the human body: major hormones and minor hormones. The major hormones have the greater role in determining what happens within your cells, and the minor hormones have the lesser role, but both major and minor hormones play a role in keeping you alive.

The major hormones are the first to be secreted in response to our constantly changing nutrition, lifestyle, and environmental signals. The major and the minor hormones communicate with each other, but the major hormones have the greater influence.

According to Dr. Schwarzbein, "The three major hormones are adrenaline, cortisol, and insulin. These hormones are crucial for life-sustaining functions such as regulating heartbeat and blood pressure and also maintaining the pH balance between blood acidity and alkalinity. So if you are missing any one of the major hormones, you will get sick quickly and not live very long. These hormones keep you alive, so there is no question as to their importance to your health and well-being." If these major hormones are low or missing, there is no controversy about whether or not to replace them. You would never deny a diabetic regular shots of insulin.

But there is a lot of controversy about replacing the minor hor-

MINOR HORMONES

ESTROGEN: Produced in the ovaries, body fat, and other parts of the body. Occurs in the body in three compounds—estradiol, estrone, and estriol. Estrogen stimulates growth in breasts, ovaries, and the uterus so the body will create eggs. Can also protect heart and brain function and promote bone strength.

PROGESTERONE: Produced primarily in the ovaries. With estrogen, progesterone prepares the lining of the uterus.

TESTOSTERONE: An androgen; produced in the ovaries and the adrenal gland. Provides sex drive.

DHEA: Made by the adrenal glands, converted into testosterone.

mones, such as estradiol, progesterone, testosterone, dehydroepi-androsterone (DHEA), and HGH (human growth hormone). Should you replace them or not? If any of the minor hormones fall too low, you will have many complaints, including fatigue, mood changes, and weight gain, but these aren't necessarily life-threatening problems. Your heart keeps beating, your blood is reasonably balanced, and your blood pressue is still within normal parameters. You are alive, but you just don't feel as well as you could if you balanced your minor hormones by replacing the ones you have lost. In *The Schwarzbein Principle II,* Dr. Schwarzbein writes, "The loss of a minor hormone will shorten your life span. However, because the loss of any one of the minor hormones does not cause immediate death, it is harder to understand their roles in sustaining health and promoting longevity."

In short her book says: "With the loss of a major hormone, you absolutely know that something is medically wrong with you, and if the major hormone is not replaced, you will die rather quickly. With the loss of a minor hormone, you will not feel well, but you are likely to attribute your health to normal aging and not seek medical attention. You will eventually die from the loss of a minor hormone, but when you die ten to fifty years later, who is to know that the minor-hormone loss contributed to your death?"

You know what Dr. Schwarzbein is talking about here by saying "normal aging"—we have all seen our mothers and their friends get older and suffer the effects of aging. We think it's normal to feel lousy when we get older—it's just something that happens when we age, right? But now that you see how important hormones are to our physiology, you can understand how vital it is to keep them balanced so we can live longer and be healthy. Because very few people understand the importance of hormones, we look for quick fixes when we start to encounter the wild fluctuations of our hormones in perimenopause and the loss of hormones in menopause. When we can't take the bad moods anymore, the irritability, the sleeplessness, and the hot flashes, we beg our doctors to take care of our symptoms, thinking that by doing this, we are taking care of the problem. Before the Women's Health Initiative (WHI) released their study in 2002 saying that HRT increased the risk of breast cancer, heart attacks, and blood clots—thus scaring many women off HRT—women thought they were finding a measure of relief in the common course of HRT, which traditionally meant prescribing Prempro, a combination of Premarin (an estrogen substitute made from pregnant mares' urine) and Provera (a progesterone substitute). But at what cost? As I explained earlier, these synthetic hormones do not in any way replace the hormones that are being lost in the body, because they are not identical to what is made in our bodies.

Drugs like Prempro do take away some of the symptoms, so there is relief and, therefore, a belief that all is well again. But then comes the weight gain—the menopausal body, as I call it. You can see the change in yourself and in your friends. Women become thicker, fuller, everywhere, with bigger arms, neck, bosom, waist, hips, legs, and butt. Where is that cute shape you once had? The clothes you once loved now fit you as though they belong to your daughter. It's hard to get dressed; nothing fits anymore. For the first time you find yourself shopping in a different department—bigger shirts, sweaters, jackets that cover the new fullness. It's depressing. You start dieting for the first time in your life. Now you are eating less, but the weight keeps coming on. Your body is not experiencing the most annoying and disturbing menopausal symptoms now, because the synthetic hormones have alleviated them, so you do not realize that your body has regrouped into survival mode to help you because it realizes that without hormones everything metabolically is starting to shut down.

Without hormones your bones also start to lose their density. So the body helps out by fattening you up to protect you in case of a fall. If you have a lot of extra padding, you might not break one of those now brittle bones. Menopausal women are the first to experience this loss, but make no mistake about it, your husbands will also experience this same phenomenon. We will talk more about this in part 4.

YOUNG WOMEN BEWARE–
YOU CAN LOSE YOUR HORMONES, TOO

Hormonal loss does not affect just menopausal women and men as they age. Younger women can also experience the loss of their hormones. Today's young woman is the new "superwoman." She does it all: has a successful business, runs the house, is the perfect mother, shows up for school events, makes cupcakes for the class, works out, gives exemplary dinner parties, sits up at night with her sick child, and so on. But stress blunts hormonal production, so this high-stress lifestyle starts to take its toll. Soon she is not looking or feeling well, her temper is out of control, she loses or gains weight, her libido shuts down, and she takes to weeping. She tries to put on an outward appearance that all is well, but it's not.

Though she may be years from menopause, the effects of stress on a young woman's body can be remarkably similar to what a woman in menopause is going through, because these young women are losing their hormones. Even younger women can benefit by temporarily replacing lost hormones due to a high-stress lifestyle and bad dietary habits. During these high-stress times a cutting-edge endocrinologist or gynecologist who understands and specializes can help by tracking hormone levels in a woman's blood work and replacing the hormones that are either high or low. Taking hormones will help you to better manage your stressful life and get things under control. It's vital to do this—stress and hormone loss will quickly age your body.

I will go into more details in chapter 4 about the medical benefits of replacing hormones. This isn't only about fighting weight gain and getting rid of hot flashes, it's also about increasing the quality and length of your life. You can't replace your declining hormone levels with synthetic hormones, *only* with bioidentical hormones. So what are these bioidentical hormones, anyway, and exactly how does a doctor figure out what a woman needs to take?

Dr. Schwarzbein has some very good advice for those who want to replace synthetic HRT with bioidentical HRT. You can read about this in her own words in the Q&A I have done with her (see chapter 5), but, in brief, she recommends you follow these four rules:

1. *Don't take a hormone that's not low or missing.*
2. *Take only bioidentical hormones.*
3. *Mimic normal physiology as much as possible.*
4. *Track the hormone levels and their effects.*

The success of this program begins with a visit to your doctor. Your doctor will monitor through blood work the hormones that need to be replaced. The goal is to try to re-create the hormonal balance experienced in your thirties (which is why I recommend that younger women get their hormone levels checked so they will know when they get older what these levels looked like in their prime). For me, it's all about trying to mimic the natural hormones I have lost, which means as I go through menopause I am low in DHEA, estradiol, and progesterone. HRT with bioidentical hormones allows us to replace our body's estrogen (called estradiol), progesterone, and testosterone (if needed) with substances that are synthesized in a lab from extracts of yam and soybeans. These hormones are not available in health food stores or from naturalists or herbalists. The bioidentical hormones are by prescription only, but they are not drugs. They are prescribed by your doctor so you can get the *exact* dosage *you* require. These bioidentical hormones exactly mimic the effects of the estradiol and progesterone that our own bodies create. You can argue that yams and soybeans are no more natural to our bodies than the pregnant mares' urine found in Premarin, an estrogen substitute, but Premarin is not synthesized to mimic exactly what our own bodies do.

Now you know, through initial blood work, which hormones need replacing. Your doctor's prescription will indicate what amounts of which hormone you need and whether you will be taking capsules, liquid, gel, or cream (different doctors prefer different ways to prescribe these hormones, based upon your needs and your ability to absorb). You can't just go to the pharmacy and buy

SYNTHETIC VS. BIOIDENTICAL HORMONES

ESTROGEN

SYNTHETIC: Premarin and other conjugated estrogens (though Premarin has dominated the market in the United States). These are derived from the urine of pregnant mares and are sometimes called "natural," but they are not natural to our bodies.

BIOIDENTICAL: Estradiol, estrone, estriol. These are synthesized in a lab from plant extracts such as soybeans and yams. Though they are created in a laboratory, they are designed molecularly to be the same as the hormones in our bodies.

PROGESTERONE

SYNTHETIC: Provera, Amen (medroxyprogesterone acetate); also norethindrone, norgestrel, and norgestimate. Prempro is a combination of Premarin and Provera.

BIOIDENTICAL: USP progesterone (Pro-Gest, Prometrium, Crinone). Extracted from a variety of wild yam, designed to be molecularly the same as the hormones in our bodies.

TESTOSTERONE

SYNTHETIC: Methyltestosterone. You can also get a combination of estradiol and synthetic testosterone called Estratest, or Premarin plus synthetic testosterone. You can get testosterone in drops, gel, patch, or cream.

BIOIDENTICAL: Dehydroepiandrosterone, or DHEA, an adrenal precursor for testosterone.

Plant-based herbs for menopausal symptoms are also available, including black cohosh and lignans for estrogen effect and chasteberry and wild yam for progesterone effect, but I got no relief from these substances.

one pill—remember, this is not a "one pill fits all" kind of therapy. You can get your dosages at compounding pharmacies, which will make preparations for you based upon your individual needs. If you don't have a compounding pharmacy in your area, I have included a list of them at the back of the book. Is this more difficult than the "one pill fits all" theory behind synthetic HRT? Absolutely, but I hope you are seeing how important it is to replace the hormones you are losing in your body with exact replicas of what has been lost, and the only way you can do that is by filling a prescription written just for you.

The goal of HRT is finding out how to mimic our physiology through the use of bioidentical hormones—it is a challenge to match the normal production and secretion of the hormone that needs to be replaced. We secrete different amounts of hormones all day long at different times of the day. If we are in a calm period, without stress, happy with our lives and relationships, maintaining a balanced HRT is rather easy. Your trip to the doctor and the results of your blood work indicate which hormones are low. Replace them in those amounts and life gets back on track. But if your life is filled with everyday stresses, compounded by deadlines and pressure, you will blunt your hormone production and your levels will change. Then it's time to call your doctor and describe the stresses you are going through. Your doctor might suggest that you "wait it out" to see if everything returns to normal—or, if that doesn't seem likely, tell you that it's time to take another blood test to see if you need to increase or decrease your levels.

This is difficult because it takes time. Most women opt for the drug hormones because there is no additional blood work and no levels to check. The "drug hormone" has only one job, and that is to take away your symptoms, but the tragedy is that nothing is being replaced. The lost hormones are gone for good. The life-sustaining nutrients supplied by your hormones are absent, and silently you begin to shut down metabolically. Aging and all that comes with it—aches, pains, weight loss or gain, disease, memory loss, and loss of mobility, agility, and libido—begin to set in.

COSTS

You may be wondering about the expense involved in using natural hormones. As a general rule, natural hormones cost around $65 a month. The first visit to your doctor costs anywhere between $100 and $300, depending upon the doctor. Usually, that is the most comprehensive and expensive appointment. After that you can do most everything else through a phone appointment with your doctor, the cost of which will vary from doctor to doctor.

Tracking your blood levels varies from person to person. With my high-stress lifestyle and the fact that I have had cancer, I usually have my blood work done every three to six months. If your lifestyle is calmer than mine, it might be as simple as having your blood work done once a year. The cost varies from lab to lab, but it is usually around $100, and it is generally covered by insurance.

Different doctors approach natural hormones in different ways. Dr. Schwarzbein, who is my personal doctor, gives natural hormones in a way that mimics normal physiology, which means I have a monthly period. My doctor administers my hormones to me in capsule form. If I have a symptom or symptoms, depending upon their severity, she prescribes a new dosage. If my symptoms are very severe, she will ask me to have blood drawn so she can see exactly where my levels are at the moment.

Dr. Uzzi Reiss administers natural hormones in liquid, gel, or cream form. When his patient is experiencing symptoms, he asks her to call him and explain the symptoms; and then he says to take more of this gel or less of that cream and check back with him to tell him whether or not the dosage works. With this technique you would probably be having blood drawn less often and, therefore, it would be less expensive.

In addition to mimicking our body's natural physiology by taking bioidentical hormones in dosages that replace exactly what our body is missing, *how* we take these hormones is important. Some doctors prescribe what is called continuous combined hormone therapy. Combined hormone therapy is taking low levels of estrogen and high levels of progesterone on a daily basis, so that your body does not get a period. Dr. Schwarzbein says, "The purpose of combined therapy was to give a woman the advantage of HRT after menopause without the uncomfortable withdrawal period. Women were actually told they had a choice, which I now know is wrong. The thinking was, take HRT and have a monthly period, or take HRT and have no uterine bleeding. Who wouldn't want the benefits of not having a period?"

Appealing as it sounds, not having a period is actually harmful, because taking hormones this way does not mimic physiology—in other words, it does not mimic the way your body used to make them. In fact, instead of decreasing the risks of certain diseases that are known to be helped by estradiol, taking HRT the wrong way increases the risk. For example, women who take combined therapy are at greater risk for heart attacks, strokes, and breast cancer. The only way to mimic the normal menstrual cycle is to take HRT and have monthly withdrawal bleeding. Taking combined therapy mimics your body's hormone balance during pregnancy, when you don't have a period (higher levels of progesterone than estradiol on a continuous basis). Postmenopausal women should not be mimicking pregnancy, since the risks associated with pregnancy (heart attack, stroke, type 2 diabetes, and breast cancer) increase exponentially with age.

Combined therapy (not having a period) can elevate levels of adrenaline, cortisol, and insulin. The longer a woman takes HRT this way, the greater her chances of burning out her adrenal glands, becoming insulin resistant, or making preexisting insulin resistance worse. If a woman's adrenal glands burn out, she increases her risk for depression, allergies, and headaches. If she becomes insulin resistant, she will increase her risk for breast cancer, blood clots, strokes, and heart attacks.

The Women's Health Initiative study from 2002 concluded after 5.2 years of follow-up that women taking Prempro (continuous combined therapy with no period) were getting more heart attacks, blood clots, strokes, and breast cancer than women who were not taking anything. The study concluded that the risks of continuous combined therapy exceeded the benefits. Even with this news, many

WATER RETENTION AND PROGESTIN

At menopausal age many women complain about water retention. Guess what? It's not a normal part of the aging process. Water retention, with very few exceptions, is caused by either too much estrogen or too little progesterone. It comes back to that same old thing: an imbalance of hormones creates imbalances in the way your body works.

Progesterone is a beautiful natural diuretic. It prevents the water retention that can be caused by estrogen. This is why combined hormone therapy is questionable. It creates imbalances. You don't have to bother with a period, but your ankles are swelling, your legs ache, your stomach is bloating, and your clothes and shoes are uncomfortable. In fact, combined therapy *increases* the risk for heart attacks, strokes, and breast cancer. The only way to mimic the normal menstrual cycle is to take HRT and have a monthly period.

Combined hormone therapy mimics your body's hormone balance during pregnancy (higher levels of progesterone than estradiol on a continuous basis). If you remember when you were pregnant, you will recall the swollen ankles and the bloated feeling you had. That is why you need to have your levels checked if you are experiencing swollen ankles. If your hormones are in balance, you'll have no fluid buildup. When I was going through radiation for my breast cancer, my hormones were being blown out by the radiation even though I was continuing to take my natural hormones. During the entire six weeks of intense radiation, and for almost a two-year period following, I was experiencing severe water retention. My ankles (which are skinny by nature) would swell up to an unrecognizable size. It took almost two years after radiation to get everything back in balance, and during this time I was reminded what it was like before I had found balance.

A new generation of progesterone substitutes, called progestins and progestogens, are being touted as the latest "natural" release from the nasty symptoms of menopause. But here's the scoop on these drugs: They cause the body to retain more fluid. The manufacturers of these products are aware that baby boomers and an increasing market of women in perimenopause and menopause are looking for a "fix" to get them through this uncomfortable life passage. But none of these products are the same as what your body makes; they have few of the protective benefits of natural progesterone and a lot of side effects and abnormal reactions.

Many qualified doctors are doing a great service to women in touting the benefits of natural progesterone and the dangers of progestins, but many physicians don't know the difference between progesterone and progestins. They haven't been trained to think about options. Some doctors don't even know that natural progesterone exists. It is your job to find out about them and to find a doctor in your area who is well versed. If your doctor is not aware of the benefits of natural hormones, perhaps you can ask him or her to read up so that the two of you can work together.

---

doctors are not warning their patients of the risks of taking HRT this way. Some even downplay the results, but taking HRT incorrectly is harmful! Dr. Schwarzbein warns, "For those who think that this study, which was done with Prempro, applies to synthetic HRT only, you are wrong. Bioidentical hormones given in a continuous combined way will be harmful because even though they are 'real' hormones, 'combined' HRT does not mimic normal physiology." Some doctors who don't understand prescribe combined natural hormone replacement so the woman does not have a period. In doing so, they are putting their patients at risk. Continuous combined natural HRT is harmful even though the hormones are natural, because daily low doses of estradiol and daily high doses of progesterone will cause the same increased risk of disease as with synthetic hormones. Adrenaline, cortisol, and insulin levels will rise higher than normal, and taking the hormones in a combined way, which does not mimic how our bodies work naturally, will increase a woman's risk for disease.*

You can gather from this information that I do not believe in continuous combined therapy. I am a firm believer in re-creating the body's natural functions. I understand that it is necessary to keep a steady stream of hormones coursing through my system continuously, throughout the day; so I take my hormones, estra-

---

* For a complete reprint of the Women's Health Initiative study, go to www.suzannesomers.com.

MY PERSONAL HRT PLAN

1. Check hormone levels with doctor through blood work.
2. Buy hormones based upon prescription at compounding pharmacy.
3. Take estradiol twice a day, every day of the month.
4. Take progesterone tenth through eighteenth day of the month.
5. Have regular checkups and additional blood work if needed to reevaluate hormone levels.

diol and progesterone, at approximately the same time each morning and the same time each night. That way I am getting closest to mimicking what my body would be doing naturally if it were still producing a full complement of hormones. I have my blood tested regularly, more often if I am experiencing a severe workload and stress. I talk with my doctor after she gets the results. We discuss any symptoms I might have and the possible reasons for them. If my blood work warrants, we increase or decrease my estradiol or progesterone.

I also take them in a cycling manner instead of taking combined continuous therapy. I take my estradiol every day of the month, but on the tenth through the eighteenth days I add the prescribed amount of progesterone. At the end of this cycle, I get a period. (Don't worry, when you are in menopause you cannot get pregnant because you no longer have eggs.) Later in this book I will talk with a few women who are in their fifties, sixties, seventies, and eighties so you can hear from them if having a period for their entire lives is worth the trade-off. I suspect it will be. You may have noticed references to another hormone, testosterone, in this chapter. In addition to estradiol and progesterone, I take testosterone, which I will talk about in chapter 9. As you know, your body works better when *all* your hormones are balanced, and you don't want to forget about this important one.

So now you understand that the hormones of the body are interconnected and one hormone imbalance leads to an imbalance of all hormones. It is very important to replace a hormone if it is low or missing and cannot be made by your body. When the body is in balance hormonally, the quality of your life will improve in every way. It truly is the "secret elixir" and the "fountain of youth." Who doesn't want that?

Perks of aging: Your secrets
are safe with your friends because they
can't remember them either.

4

FINDING THE RIGHT DOCTOR

What is the difference between young people and older people? It's vitality. Vitality is strength, vigor, excitement, curiosity, stamina, energy, a feeling of being "on the ball"! Vitality is something you radiate, it's something from within—a natural zest for life.

We don't entirely lose our vitality as we age, but in our middle years we become aware that we no longer have the kind of energy we once had. "Let the young people handle it, they have all the energy," we moan. Do you want to feel the way you did when you were young? You know the answer—get your hormones balanced!

It is my belief that in the near future the medical community will understand what we passionate laypersons and cutting-edge doctors already know: We need to balance our lost hormones by replacing them with natural bioidentical hormones that mimic what our bodies created when we were in our prime. And why not? If the medical community is so intent upon keeping us alive until we are ninety to one hundred years old, then let's make sure those last twenty or twenty-five "extra years" are quality ones. By eating right, exercising, thinking good thoughts, avoiding chemicals, moderating alcohol intake, and eliminating smoking, you are on track. Add balanced hormones to this scenario, and wow! These last "extra years" could be your best.

What most people don't understand is that recent reports offering negative statistics about hormone replacement therapy are based upon research conducted on synthetic (drug) hormones. Most of the studies that extol the benefits of synthetic hormones are funded by the drug companies that make them. Natural hormones are not patentable, so the drug companies are not interested in them—there's no profit margin. Don't be angry, it's just business. But it's up to you to be proactive. If you want a better quality of life, it's up to you to find out all you can about options.

As I've said, when we are young our bodies produce a full complement of hormones. They keep us young and supple, agile, lubricated, sexual. Because we are living longer than ever before, the new thinking is to *replace* the hormones lost in the aging process. This *cannot* be done with the synthetic hormones put out by the drug companies; drug hormones can eliminate most of the physical symptoms of hormone loss, but they do *not replace hormones* lost in the aging process. Only natural bioidentical hormones can do that, because they are made from plant extracts and exactly mimic the hormones we make naturally in our bodies.

It is extremely difficult to find a doctor to concur with this way of thinking. Most doctors (good ones) are influenced by drug companies. They are given those free samples we all love to get when we go to the doctor's office, and then the literature and studies that are fed to doctors from the drug companies become "fact," when in many cases they have little to do with what will really heal us. Drugs in general do not heal; they abate and remove pain. Let me say again, I would not like to live in a world without pharmaceuticals. I simply feel that drugs should always be our last resort.

As I mentioned earlier, I went from doctor to doctor to get to the bottom of this "mysterious passage." I was frustrated by the answers I was getting. It wasn't until I found an endocrinologist who specialized in bioidentical HRT that I finally got some satisfaction. Frankly, "satisfaction" is not a strong enough word; "bliss" would be more apt.

As I also mentioned earlier, in medical school our doctors get approximately four hours of training in the study of hormones. How can a doctor, even a gynecologist, be an "expert" with so little training? That is why I prefer to get my information from someone who has made the study of menopause, and andropause (male menopause), his or her specialty. Generally this is the domain of endocrinologists, but there are gynecologists and other doctors who have continued their studies and their interest in the phenomenon of natural bioidentical hormones. Finding this blissful balance is the best thing I have done for myself at this passage. I want to be involved with doctors who are forward thinking and well versed in the hormonal system. This is no time for guessing. It is too important to my well-being. I love my life, and I want to get the most out of it.

It can be very hard to find someone to help you. Finding the right doctor is difficult. Your gynecologist may not be the right person for you at this time. Menopause and hormones should be his or her specialty if you are being treated for a possible hormonal deficiency as you approach middle age. If it is not your gynecologist's specialty, then you have to find a doctor who "gets it." A gynecologist who is not well versed in the hormonal system, who is trying to treat you for menopause with synthetic hormones or claims to know about natural hormones and then gives you a prescription without requiring a blood test, is not going to be able to help you; it would be like asking your dermatologist to perform open heart surgery. It's not enough to simply know where the heart is located—the doctor must know everything about the heart and how it works. If your doctor claims to be a hormone specialist, ask about his or her credentials. This is too important—you have to ask questions.

Balancing your hormones takes knowledge, and the only professionals I am aware of who have the information to do this are endocrinologists and doctors who have made the study of natural bioidentical hormones their specialty. Even endocrinologists need to be asked if they are well versed in natural bioidentical hormones, because not all of them are up on the latest advances. Maybe when they were in school the information was not available yet, or maybe they never kept up with the latest advances. So it is up to you to scour your community to find the right professional. If you have to travel to another city to find a competent endocrinologist or specialist, believe me, it's worth the trip. Just make sure you're seeing a qualified M.D. and not an herbalist or a naturalist. You want a studied professional to treat you during this tricky passage. This is about the quality of your life. There is no reason to suffer. But without the right advice and program, you will, indeed, suffer through this passage and your health will gradually go downhill.

I prefer a female endocrinologist only because this is a female syndrome and I feel that a woman might have a better understanding than a male doctor; but again, there are always exceptions. Dr. Uzzi Reiss, a gynecologist, has made natural hormones his specialty, and he is kind, caring, understanding, and sensitive

WHAT YOU NEED TO KNOW
WHEN YOU GO TO THE DOCTOR

1. Ask to get your baseline hormone levels checked in a lab (you need to have estradiol, progesterone, and follicle-stimulating hormone [FSH] checked).

2. Tell your doctor you want to be prescribed bioidentical estradiol and progesterone.

3. Ask your doctor to recommend a good compounding pharmacy that will combine the proper amounts of estradiol and progesterone based upon the doctor's prescription (go to the Resources in the back of the book if you don't have a compounding pharmacy in your area).

4. When you get your preparations, you will probably take your estradiol twice a day, about twelve hours apart, and one progesterone pill for fourteen days of each month—the easiest way to do this is days one to fourteen. Cycling this way mimics your body's natural production of hormones. Your dosages should be monitored by a physician, but you will most likely start with about .5 mg of estradiol twice a day, with 100 mg of progesterone a day.

5. You will get your period around the time you stop taking progesterone. If you bleed early, you may be taking either too much progesterone or not enough estradiol and you need your blood levels checked again.

about women's health and this passage in particular. It is difficult for anyone to grasp the effects physically, psychologically, and emotionally of losing 90 percent of your hormones over a two-year period, but some male physicians are able to do so.

It's a simple fact that one cannot have a satisfactory life if one doesn't have satisfactory hormones. Hormones are the body's very own all-natural antiaging pill. And what a pill! Women who are afraid or confused about hormones will unfortunately experience the negative consequences of not taking them. How about rotting bones, dried-up vaginal tissue, droopy breasts, skin with no elasticity, a double chance of Alzheimer's disease, and double or triple the likelihood that sooner or later a heart attack will finish the story? That's just part of it.

Dr. Eugene Shippen, another of our country's leading endocrinologists, says, "There are astonishing advantages of hormone replacement in women. Nothing in medicine has been studied so intensively for so many years and through so many patient trials and investigations as estrogen replacement therapy. Nothing generates more controversy, phobic reactions, and confusion. Yet surprisingly, it would be hard to find a treatment in which an amazing long-term success rate is combined with so few side effects. The advantages of giving estrogen so far outweigh the risks that rational opposition to postmenopausal hormone replacement in women is very difficult to sustain. The therapy's ability to offer women aging modification, disease prevention, and improved quality of life is so remarkable and has been replicated so repeatedly in medical studies that it's sometimes hard to know what all the controversy is about."

As women, we get around forty years of life, from puberty to menopause, in which to enjoy the health-promoting benefits of estrogen. During this time we experience the life-giving benefits that come from making a full complement of hormones. When we are young, we are our healthiest. Heart attacks and strokes barely exist when we are premenopausal. Arthritis is rare; our immune systems are outstanding. It is not until after menopause that things start to go wrong. The acceleration toward poor health that then occurs in so many women's bodies is not coincidental in the slightest. It is hormonal to the core. Postmenopausally, without our hormones, we women lose the major programmer of our health.

Over the age of fifty-five, approximately 48 percent of all women die of cardiovascular disease, principally heart attacks and strokes. Twenty-four percent of us die from some form of cancer, 1.5 percent of which is breast cancer. Hormone replacement (real hormone replacement) is found in most studies to reduce the rate of death from cardiovascular disease by 30 to 40 percent, a drop in total mortality of approximately 14 to 19 percent. Meanwhile, worst-case projections show an increase in breast cancer of 10 percent, which would represent a total mortality increase of .15 percent. The cost-benefit ratio turns out to be almost fantastically skewed in favor of hormone replacement. The choice remains a very individual one for us, but based upon personal risk factors, the meaning of these statistics seems clear.

I'll say it once again (and again and again and again): Balancing hormones is our best bet to fight the diseases of aging. Upon middle age (the menopausal passage), we begin to get our first reports of high blood pressure, plaque in our arteries, diabetes, weight gain, and personality changes. Balanced hormones are our best defense against disease. It is not normal to get sick as we age. But without balanced hormones, our organs are not getting the proper nutrients and begin slowly to break down. It is commonly thought that middle age brings sickness. In general it does because there is so little understanding of hormone replacement.

I cannot tell you how great I feel when my hormones are in balance. I spend the time it takes to achieve this balance, despite my superbusy schedule, because it is my belief that an environment of balanced hormones prevents disease. I believe this so firmly that I am relying on balanced hormones as a means to fight my breast cancer. I believe this is my edge over this disease. This is my personal belief, and I am not recommending that you do as I do. I simply state my opinion as a means of conveying to you how strongly I believe in HRT.

But I am not alone. Studies show that the total improvement in life expectancy when women remain on natural bioidentical estrogen replacement is more than significant. In 1966, a study was conducted by Dr. Bruce Ettinger, who followed five hundred women who belonged to the Kaiser Permanente health system in California. Two hundred and thirty-two of these women were on bioidentical estrogen replacement for an average of seventeen years, compared with 222 women who had been on estrogen for an average of less than one year during the same period. It was discovered that the death rate from all causes was lower by 44 percent in the women on estrogen for seventeen years. Remember, I am talking about natural bioidentical hormones, not drug hormones. But it begs one question: Why is the death rate so much lower for women on estrogen?

Did you know that men have significantly larger arteries than women, and because of this, it is easier for women's arteries to become blocked? Did you know that heart disease is the biggest single killer of women as well as men? Dr. Shippen says: "According to the current evidence, if not for hormones, women would be significantly more at risk for heart attacks and strokes than men. Men get heart attacks sooner, even though testosterone gives them protection; but it does not compare with the protection that hormones give to women. Once postmenopausal women lose their hormonal protection, in less than fifteen years they begin to have heart attacks as fast as men. Yet in women who replace estrogen, this change does not occur."

The *New England Journal of Medicine* conducted a study on five thousand women who were taking estrogen. It concluded, based upon improvements in their risk factors, that they would experience a 42 percent reduction in their rate of heart disease. British researchers, analyzing their own data, came up with a figure of 50 percent. According to Dr. Shippen, women who take real hormones that are balanced have:

higher levels of good HDL cholesterol.

lower levels of bad LDL cholesterol.

lower levels of fibrinogen.

lower levels of plasminogen activator inhibitor-1 (PAI-1).

lower levels of homocysteine.

lower levels of insulin.

lower levels of glucose.

lower levels of lipoprotein (a).

increases in blood flow to all parts of the body, including the brain, heart, muscles, skin, and bones.

Now what does this mean to you and me? Well . . . here's the science: HDL cholesterol, the "good" cholesterol, transports LDL out of the tissues and back to the liver for excretion.

LDL cholesterol, the "bad" cholesterol, triggers the activity of large cells that engulf bacteria and unwanted debris, including particles of LDL. The engorged cells then become foam cells, and these trigger changes in the walls of the artery leading to plaque formation.

Fibrinogen is a natural clot-forming substance in the bloodstream. High levels of fibrinogen make it more likely that a blockage in a major artery will result in a heart attack.

Plasminogen activator inhibitor-1 (PAI-1) decreases the body's ability to inhibit the formation of blood clots. It increases the likelihood that complete blockage of an artery will precipitate a heart attack.

Homocysteine derives from methionine, an essential amino acid that is found in fairly high levels in the American diet. Estrogen helps to lower homocysteine levels and has significant lifesaving effects.

Insulin and glucose are significantly lowered by taking estrogen.

Lipoprotein is a type of cholesterol that is a particularly high risk for heart attack. It turns out that estrogen is one of the few substances that can effectively lower it.

It is misleading to women of menopausal age to have the medical community continue to put out flawed negative reports on HRT. Women are terribly confused, and no wonder why. The reports that create such alarm and cause such a media frenzy are done on "drug hormones," which contain very little in the way of hormones at all, but are simply "symptom suppressors." So certainly women taking drug hormones are having heart attacks, heart disease, high blood pressure, diabetes, strokes, Alzheimer's, and a host of other diseases. If drug hormones are simply taking away the uncomfortable symptoms of menopause, but not replacing the hormones lost in the aging process, a woman would be left open to a whole host of diseases because she has no protection. As I said before, it is an environment of balanced hormones that prevents disease.

Hormones are your protection—real hormones such as estradiol, progesterone, and testosterone are identical to the hormones found in the human body. Drugs like conjugated estrogens (Premarin), medroxyprogesterone acetate (Provera), and methyltestosterone are chemicals not found in the human body. In other words, they can't do the job properly. They will lull you into a false sense of well-being. Because you are not experiencing the miserable symptoms of menopause, you'll think all is okay again, but the organs and systems of the body are breaking down and there is nothing to build them back up. Before you know it, disease sets in.

Signs of menopause: You have to write
Post-it notes with your kids' names on them.

5

DR. DIANA SCHWARZBEIN:
MENOPAUSE

For any of you who have read any of my books on Somersizing, you know the important role Dr. Schwarzbein plays in my life. She is an awesome doctor, cutting-edge, and the first doctor I met who truly understands menopause and its ramifications. As an endocrinologist, her specialty is the chemical makeup of the body. As I struggled to find a doctor who really understood what my body was going through in menopause (before I found the wonderful doctors I have interviewed for this book), it was Dr. Schwarzbein who was finally able to help me find relief. She understands the importance of replacing the hormones lost in the aging process with natural hormones that are exact replicas (bioidentical) of the ones we make in our own bodies. Because of Dr. Schwarzbein, I am enjoying my menopause more than any other passage so far. Here is our conversation.

SS: First of all, I appreciate your giving me time to do this. I know how swamped you are at the office.

Every woman is looking for answers during this confusing passage, and you have made menopause a specialty. So let me first ask you: Because menopause is confusing not only to women but also to most doctors, how did you figure it out?

DS: Most of what I know about hormone replacement therapy in menopause I did not learn in medical school, or in medical training. It was when I was in private practice. I had four years of medical school, three years of internal medicine, then two years of endocrinology, but in nine years of training no one said, This is menopause, this is what you need to be doing.

SS: What made you pay attention?

DS: I started treating diabetic patients back in 1991, and I was noticing that a subset of my diabetic patients who happened to be menopausal women, who were following the exact same diet and exercise program as all the other diabetic patients, were not responding with the same good results. In other words, their sugars were not budging. It was startling. They were eating the same way, doing the same kinds of exercises, but their blood sugars were staying at 300, whereas the men and the premenopausal women had blood sugar levels that were coming down.

SS: What were you missing?

DS: It started to dawn on me that maybe the sex hormones were playing a role in their problem. But initially I made a lot of mistakes.

SS: For instance?

DS: If someone said to you, you can have all the benefits of hormone replacement therapy with or without a period, everyone would probably say, "Oh, without a period, please."

SS: Very understandable. I mean, who wants to have a period if they don't have to?

DS: I agree, and at that point I bought into the current standard of care that believed you could have the benefits of hormones without a period. But I found that when you give hormones that way [continuously combining an estrogen with a progestin on a daily basis], you make the patient more insulin resistant.

SS: But isn't a woman her healthiest when she is pregnant, because her body is making estrogen and progesterone simultaneously?

DS: Actually, no. Pregnancy is not the healthiest state for a woman to be in. In fact, pregnancy is one of the times when you are more insulin resistant. If you are pregnant back to back and you have many children, I guarantee you're going to end up with type 2 diabetes or another form of insulin resistance such as obesity, abnormal cholesterol levels, and/or high blood pressure. Also, we now realize that pregnant women have a higher risk of breast cancer.

SS: Why is that?

DS: I am not sure that anybody really knows, but I'm going to say I think it's because of insulin resistance. Because high insulin levels have been linked to breast cancer. For instance, women with type 2 diabetes have one of the highest risks of developing breast cancer. So do women with metabolic syndrome [an insulin-resistant problem].

SS: Okay, but why would pregnancy make you insulin resistant?

DS: It's complex, but to simplify, physiologically you have many hormonal changes in pregnancy that block the action of insulin. One of them is the high progesterone levels.

SS: But people always think of pregnancy as a high estrogen state.

DS: Actually, pregnancy produces high estrogen levels but much *higher* daily progesterone levels, and the progesterone blocks the action of estrogen every day. The result of this is a low estrogen effect in the body.

SS: So let's get back to how you started treating your diabetic menopausal patients.

DS: I started treating women with diabetes in 1991, and I prescribed Prempro to those who were in menopause. Luckily, I noticed right away that their blood sugar control worsened. This was a group of patients who were not improving despite how hard they were working at eating well and exercising. In fact, some of them were getting worse. That's when I realized Prempro was the problem. Then I switched these women to estradiol and progesterone, thinking the bioidentical hormones would be the answer. However, I still prescribed them in a continuous combined way (no periods), and their blood sugars remained elevated.

Then I thought about the four rules that I use for the replacement of any missing hormone:

1. *Don't take a hormone that's not low or missing.*

2. *Take only bioidentical hormones.*
3. *Mimic normal physiology as much as possible.*
4. *Track the hormone levels and their effects.*

Starting with rule number one—in menopause you are low in estradiol and progesterone. Rule number two, give back the same hormone in its bioidentical form. I realized that Premarin was being substituted for estradiol, and Provera was being substituted for progesterone, and this was not the right thing to do. So I prescribed bioidentical estradiol for estradiol and bioidentical progesterone for progesterone.

Then, because of rule number three, I realized that continuous combined therapy was not the way the body made these hormones. To mimic normal physiology as much as possible, these hormones would have to be taken in a cyclical manner, and then women would have to have withdrawal menses [monthly period] again.

Then, rule number four, I followed my patients by tracking their hormone levels through blood work and the effects of these bioidentical hormones.

When I followed my four rules of hormone replacement that I used in treating all types of hormone deficiencies, the blood sugars of the women with diabetes improved and their hormone levels came back into balance. Finally, these women felt well again.

I realized the mistake I was making [ten years ago] treating menopausal women with type 2 diabetes was in giving them continuous combined HRT. Remember, as diabetics they were already insulin resistant, and they became more insulin resistant on continuous combined HRT. Unfortunately, many doctors today still don't understand the link between continuous combined therapy and insulin resistance and are still making the same mistake today that I did all those years ago.

In my opinion, the harm of continuous combined therapy was confirmed in July 2002, when the first results of the Women's Health Initiative was published. There were three groups of women in this study:

1. *The observational group. These women were in menopause but*

were given only a placebo. They were "observed" to check for heart disease, breast cancer, stroke, blood clots, type 2 diabetes, and so forth.

2. *Two treatment groups: subdivided by whether the woman had a uterus or did not because of a hysterectomy.*

If the woman had a uterus, she was given Prempro, a synthetic drug hormone comprising an estrogen, Premarin, and a progestin, Provera. Progestins block the effect of estrogen, so the women on Prempro did not get a period. In other words, if you take an estrogen and then block the action of it with a progestin, you end up with a low estrogen effect in the body. Hence, no bleeding.

If she didn't have a uterus, she was given Premarin alone. [Premarin is a drug that contains many different estrogens, most of which are not found or made in the human body.] Taking Premarin alone would lead to a higher estrogen effect in the body.

SS: Interesting. And when you have a low estrogen effect because of continuous combined HRT [no period], are you subject to disease?

DS: That's what the WHI study showed. It was going to be an eight-plus-year study. They wanted to compare the outcome of the treatment groups with those of the observational group.

But at 5.2 years, the Prempro study was stopped early.

SS: Why?

DS: They started noticing that the women on Prempro [continuous combined therapy—no period] were having more heart attacks, more strokes, more blood clots, and more breast cancer than the group taking the placebo.

SS: What about the women who were taking Premarin?

DS: They haven't found the same kind of increased risk for disease with Premarin alone; therefore, that part of the WHI study is still ongoing. It is slated to be finished and reported in 2005 after eight years plus.

Last year when the news broke out about Prempro, the initial reaction was to get all women off all HRT, and to this day that is what most physicians are recommending.

SS: Why was the Women's Health Initiative done in the first place?

DS: The idea was to do a long-term prospective study on the possible benefits versus risks of the most commonly used HRT. They studied Premarin and Prempro because these are the most commonly prescribed therapies.

SS: So, when a woman takes these drug hormones, is she getting any good out of it at all, or would she be better off not taking anything?

DS: The WHI concluded that Prempro is worse than not taking anything, and I agree with the conclusion.

SS: That's a pretty strong statement.

DS: Yes, but that's what the study concluded.

As far as Premarin goes, I do not like it because it is not a bioidentical estrogen. However, it hasn't been shown to be more harmful than not taking anything at all. But this part of the study is still ongoing. It's important to know that Premarin has not yet been shown to be of much benefit, either. When it first came on the market, it was only supposed to be used in the short term to treat hot flashes, but then its use got extended (without any studies, I might add) to long-term hormone replacement therapy for menopause. As far as I am concerned, one of the uses of HRT after menopause should be for protection against heart disease. Premarin does not protect against heart disease.

SS: Well, all I know is I am feeling so wonderful that I am going to take bioidentical [natural] hormones for life, or as long as I choose to do so.

DS: And I believe it is safe for you to take bioidentical hormones for the rest of your life as long as we keep monitoring the effects of these hormones and we keep adjusting the amount to match your ever-changing lifestyle.

SS: Now what about Prempro or Premarin? Would a gynecologist put a woman on these drugs for life?

DS: I know many women who have been on these drugs for too long. There are two paralleling concepts going on: One is don't substitute a drug for a hormone; they do not do the same thing in the body. Two, do not think that you are going to come up with a better way to give these drugs than to match the physiology that already exists, as in natural bioidentical hormones.

I learned from my own studies and my treatment of menopausal women that you can approach menopause in two ways: symptomatic relief therapy or bioidentical HRT following the four rules mentioned earlier. Most gynecologists have been approaching it from the symptomatic side. They feel that as long as a woman is not having hot flashes, she is being treated properly. That is not true.

Furthermore, in my experience most gynecologists treat the uterus as the most important organ in the human body. As such, they feel their role is to keep harm from coming to your uterus. The medical literature in gynecology is filled with studies on the amount of progestin needed to protect the uterus from developing cancer. In trying to save the uterus and prescribing continuous combined therapy, gynecologists have increased the risk of breast cancer, heart attacks, and strokes in once-healthy women! Unfortunately, by messing with Mother Nature and giving drug hormones without restoring menstrual bleeding, we have done more harm than good.

SS: Okay, here we are again at having a period.

DS: You have to have a period, because this mimics normal! The normal state is not pregnancy! Prempro mimics pregnancy, so continuous combined therapy is *not* normal. Having a monthly period is normal. At one point gynecologists understood this concept. Prior to the last ten to fifteen years, most doctors did prescribe Premarin and Provera in a cycling way. That was the standard of care for quite some time.

SS: Then what happened?

DS: Primarily, women weren't feeling good on Premarin and Provera. They were complaining of bloating and irritability and on top of it were getting their period again! Then many women stopped taking HRT because they felt so poorly on it. Instead of treating women with bioidentical hormones, gynecologists tried different ways to give Provera to protect against uterine cancer and came up with continuous combined therapy without thinking about or studying the long-term consequences.

SS: Quite a dilemma. So if rule number three is to mimic normal physiology as much as possible, that would mean having a period, but is having a period *all your life* normal?

DS: Medically we are altering natural phenomena everywhere. There is nothing natural about immunizations, or open heart surgery, or hip replacement surgery. We have to decide as a society whether we are all going to honor aging or not. If we are, then I would say don't give hormone replacement therapy. But if as a society we choose to alter natural phenomena medically, we have to be consistent. Taking HRT after menopause is not natural, but neither is performing open heart surgery.

SS: Let's talk more about rule number four—tracking.

DS: Tracking means monitoring the effect of the hormone a woman is taking. It is done through assessing hormone levels, assessing how the woman feels on hormones, when and how much bleeding she has on a monthly basis, assessing bones and cholesterol, and evaluating her uterine lining with yearly ultrasounds. It also entails following specific issues pertinent to the woman's personal health history such as blood pressure, insulin, and blood sugar levels.

Menopause is a serious condition. In other words, I don't just prescribe hormones and say, "Have a nice life, call me if you get a hot flash." Menopause needs to be followed just like any other hormone replacement therapy. Dosages of hormones may need to be continuously adjusted around a woman's aging and her changing lifestyle.

SS: What about self-medicating, as in today my breasts are a little more tender, I think I'll take a little more estrogen cream?

DS: I don't feel very comfortable with women self-medicating around symptoms. For instance, let's take breast tenderness . . . it could be from too little estrogen or too much estrogen. So how would a woman know what to do?

I'll tell you something else about estrogen: It can act like an anti-depressant, and women can end up taking too much of it if left to determine how much they should be on in relation to how they feel. Then you get into the complications of high hormone effect in the system.

And then there is progesterone. Women cannot tell if they're taking too much progesterone because it is a stimulant and can initially make one feel better. It isn't until later that they can start feeling depressed or gain weight from too much progesterone, and by then they may not realize it's the progesterone because of how long it took before the symptoms occurred.

SS: Oh, so that is why you don't like women to self-adjust their hormones.

DS: Right, you have to be very careful. You do not want too much or too little. It has to be just right, and the only way to do that is through tracking.

SS: Should women and men go only to an endocrinologist who specializes in bioidentical HRT to get their sex hormones balanced?

DS: As an endocrinologist, I have chosen to specialize in sex hormones. But not every endocrinologist has the same training. I wish I could say, "Go to your local endocrinologist and everything will be okay." Unfortunately each person must find the right endocrinologist or doctor for him- or herself. It will require interviewing the doctor to see if he or she has made sex hormones a specialty.

SS: When you do get your hormones in balance (as you have helped me balance mine), life is blissful. It's worth a trip or a drive to another city to get on track. After all, it is a three-hour drive for me to see you, but you are worth it.

DS: Well, thank you. Now that you and I have worked together for all these years, you know that hormone replacement therapy can be complex.

SS: And this is where the concept of synthetic pharmaceutical hormones is screwy to me. How *can* one pill fit all?

DS: Exactly. Even though we all share the same physiology, we don't all share the same metabolism rate of different hormones. I mean, you and I have completely different body types. Let's look in the mirror at ourselves: Who has more estrogen . . . you or me?

SS: Old friendly me. Curvy body . . . you get to have a long, lean body and slim hips (I hate you, by the way). But I get your point. Every "body" has different needs.

DS: It's also genetics. It's about ratios among different hormones.

SS: Right now the ratio, the match, you have prescribed for me feels good. I'm feeling fantastic.

DS: Great. But it's sometimes a very difficult thing to find the perfect match for women. It takes patience and focus.

SS: How difficult?

DS: Well, it depends on their lifestyle and what is going on.

SS: So if a woman lived by a river and didn't work and didn't have a telephone or a television set and wasn't constantly thinking, Oh, my God, I have to juggle a million things . . .

DS: It would be easier to find a match for that woman. She could probably get away with much less estrogen, because estrogen is the multitasking hormone. But if this same woman smoked, it would make the body rid itself of the estradiol faster.

Another example is you, Suzanne, when you were going through that period where you were so stressed. Your hormone needs kept going up, so I had to keep changing your doses, yet your hormone levels stayed the same, because you were using it up so much. And then abruptly your stress stopped and the dose of your hormones was too much for you. All of a sudden you had a high estrogen effect.

SS: Right, and that was excessive bleeding . . .

DS: Yes, you called me and I decreased your doses and things got on track and in balance again.

SS: What's interesting to me as the patient who has been doing this for several years is that I have become very sensitive to when the doses are not correct. I find this an incredible way to work with you as my doctor. We are doing this in concert together, and it helps me to feel that I am in control of my health and my body.

DS: Yes, and as you recall when we first started working together, I was very clear about the fact that this is a pain in the butt. A "one pill fits all" would be a lot easier, but the rewards of doing it this way, from a health standpoint, a quality-of-life standpoint, and a longevity standpoint, are indisputable.

And it's not just about the hormones. It's about eating well and stress management, and tapering off sugar and other chemicals, and doing the right kinds of exercise. All hormones talk to one another. So you can't take estradiol and progesterone and expect to find balance if your insulin and adrenaline levels are going crazy from poor nutrition and lifestyle habits. Every hormone has to be in balance with the other hormones.

SS: That makes a lot of sense. A woman has to have better habits after menopause to keep her hormones in balance to help keep her prescribed hormones in balance, too. How do you feel about gynecologists giving antidepressants to quell menopausal symptoms?

DS: I think it's a tragedy. We are one of the first generations of women to fully experience this passage. We have much higher stress levels and more anxiety in our lives than ever before, and we are seeing menopause at earlier ages. And all this accelerated aging is due to bad lifestyle and dietary habits! Giving a woman an antidepressant to deal with the suffering of menopause does nothing to replace the hormones she has lost in the aging process. Antidepressants take away the vibration of living and create a host of other problems. Menopause is natural, but dying is natural also! Today we have ways of dealing effectively with menopause or delaying death; why wouldn't we want to take correct advantage of that? Antidepressants are not the answer.

SS: So what is the answer?

DS: Remember this concept . . . she who keeps her hormone levels highest the longest wins. That's the race, dear!

It's got to start with good nutrition. People don't realize that if they want to be busy and run around like a crazy person, and they don't eat well, then they will literally eat themselves!

If a woman of childbearing age wants to make a baby but is

under any type of stress, she can end up dealing with infertility. Eggs are dispensable. This is not the time to make a baby, because she needs to use whatever she would use to make an egg for energy instead to fight off the stress.

We have advanced medically so that women no longer need to die prematurely from childbirth or from infectious diseases as they did before we had antibiotics. Women also used to die in peri-menopause from infections before proper medicine was available, because we are more susceptible to infections during this phase. Women are their healthiest and strongest during their childbearing years, when they are making a full complement of hormones. The loss of hormones makes you weak.

SS: So the theory is that if I keep my hormones balanced and I continue to eat right, I can expect to stay strong and most likely avoid the diseases of aging?

DS: Right, and we now know that it's not just about menopause. It's about nutrition and stress management and sleep and exercise, and hormone replacement, if needed.

SS: Are we baby boomers the guinea pigs?

DS: I think the women who have been given the chemicals are the bigger guinea pigs. Come on, giving drugs to replace a hormone? These chemicals will cause you to lose the hormones that protect you from heart disease, namely estradiol. Real hormones provide protection from heart disease if given in bioidentical form [exact replicas of the hormones we make in our own bodies]. This was confirmed by the Howard Hodis study at the University of Southern California. He showed that estradiol—not Premarin, not synthetic hormones, not drugs, but the bioidentical estradiol found in human ovaries—will protect a woman against heart disease.

SS: Okay, Dr. Schwarzbein, we're sold, but where am I going to send women to find this kind of excellence and understanding relative to this passage? Women are barraged with bad medical advice and are highly influenced by the drug companies, so where do they go, and what should they ask their own doctor? For instance, the woman says, "I am in menopause, I am having hot flashes, I am irritable, and I am bloating."

DS: First thing to ask your doctor is to get baseline hormone levels through lab work. You want to have your estradiol, progesterone, and follicle-stimulating-hormone levels tested. If you are in menopause, you proceed to rule two.

Tell your doctor that you want to be prescribed bioidentical estradiol and progesterone. You can get the best form of these hormones from a good compounding pharmacy. Next, ask your doctor if he or she knows or works with a good compounding pharmacy. If not, or if you don't have one in your area, have them check the reference guide you have provided in the back of this book. However, some doctors won't know how to use the compounding pharmacy, so ask them to prescribe an estradiol preparation such as Estrace or Gynodiol found in the local pharmacies. There is also a noncompounded form of bioidentical progesterone known as Prometrium.

SS: How would someone know how much to take?

DS: You always want to take the lowest dose and taper up slowly.

SS: And see how you feel?

DS: Yes, and take the estradiol hormone twice a day. Estradiol is in and out of the body very quickly, so you really need to take smaller amounts more frequently to achieve the best balance. Take it twice a day about twelve hours apart, because you want to mimic a steady stream, as if your own body is still making it. The progesterone may be taken once a day or sometimes twice a day if needed.

SS: Okay, they have their estradiol and progesterone preparations. Now what?

DS: They will need to take them in a cycling manner. Take the estradiol every day of the month twice a day and add in one pill of progesterone for fourteen days out of each month. The easiest way to do this is on calendar days one through fourteen of every month.

SS: What dosage should they take?

DS: Start with about 0.5 mg of estradiol twice a day and with 100 mg of progesterone a day, and then track symptoms and levels to determine if a higher or lower dose is needed.

SS: What happens after the fourteenth day of progesterone? Is that when a woman should expect to have her period?

DS: Yes, they are supposed to be having a regular menstrual flow around the end of the progesterone or just after it is finished. . . . If they break through early [bleeding], then they are taking either too much progesterone or not enough estradiol.

SS: How will they know?

DS: They will need to have their blood levels checked to see which one it is.

Now, we are not taking into account that some people would like to be on progesterone 50 mg twice a day, not 100 mg once a day. Unfortunately, we don't have a 50 mg at every drugstore. We only have 100 mg. You have to try to work with it. But if you are able to work with a compounding pharmacy, they will be able to work it out to fit your needs more specifically.

SS: This will be a big help to women who are frustrated and do not live in an area that has an informed endocrinologist or gynecologist. As women, we have to be proactive about our health and our hormonal needs, because there is so much misinformation and lack of understanding about this passage. That is the point of this book, to empower women and men (and believe me, they also lose their hormones) to find quality health care and information about hormones for themselves.

DS: We are in a crisis as far as menopause is concerned. Doctors are going to have to learn something new, because we can't keep allowing women to suffer and become ill due to the lack of understanding that exists.

SS: So what is the future? I agree with you that menopause is a crisis at this time with this lack of understanding among women and doctors, but another generation is coming up right after us, and everyone is still in a state of confusion and frustration. Women my age are suffering, their marriages are falling apart, the divorce rate is going up, men are remarrying young girls to get the fun back in their lives, so what is going to happen? What are your hopes?

DS: Menopausal women have to demand answers. We also have to get them over their fear of breast cancer and of estrogen. One of my hopes is that the right information gets out. Women have to know that the risk of breast cancer is much less than the risk of dying from not taking hormones, or the risk of getting a heart attack or a debilitating stroke.

Let me state that insulin is a much bigger hormone relative to breast cancer than estrogen will ever be, because insulin is a major growth hormone. Insulin is a major growth hormone and estradiol is a minor growth hormone. Breast cancer is not caused because you took estradiol. Breast cancer comes from damage to DNA from the environment and damage caused by unhealthy lifestyle and dietary habits.

SS: Like . . .

DS: Stress, smoking, too much caffeine, high daily doses of progestins, lots of artificial sugar, anything that you put in your body that shouldn't be there. If you damage an area of the DNA that promotes a tumor, then that tumor is going to start to grow. Estradiol is a growth factor for normal breast tissue. So if you have normal breast tissue, but now the DNA of that normal breast tissue gets damaged, estradiol is still going to make it grow, but it didn't cause the damage.

In fact, I am going to stick my neck out and say that when we finally get around to studying bioidentical estradiol, it is going to be shown to be protective against cancers because it is an antioxidant in the human body.

Again, though, it is not about too much or too little of a hormone. The balance has to be just right.

SS: Thank you so much.

Signs of menopause: You sell your home heating system at a yard sale.

6

MARTA: A FORTY-FIVE-YEAR-OLD EXPERIENCE

Marta is a successful television producer of megahit sitcoms, a mother of three, busy from morning until night, and she has one foot in the menopausal door. But she has not hit the wall yet; she has symptoms that come and go, and her life is extremely stressful just trying to keep it all together. She has recently begun to dabble in natural hormones, and here is what she had to say about it. . . .

SS: Obviously, menopause is right around the corner for you. You are forty-five, and this is one condition no one escapes, so how are you feeling?

MK: I'm not sure how I am feeling, but I go to Dr. Uzzi Reiss and he is amazing. He is a women's health advocate. He told me I am an estrogen type, meaning that my body makes a lot of estrogen. Normally, he said, a doctor might look at my estrogen levels and say, "You are not perimenopausal," but Dr. Reiss said that the dip in my estrogen levels is so enormous, even though I still make a lot of it, that I need to replace what I am losing. I like him because he takes you as an individual.

SS: So are you feeling better being on replacement?

MK: My problem is I have such a thing about medication of any kind, including homeopathic and holistic, that I react to doing anything daily.

SS: So Dr. Reiss is giving you hormones because your ratios are

off, but you don't always take them. How long does it take before
your symptoms start to reappear?

MK: Basically, I don't even notice it until the week before my
period, and then I find myself crying because my coffee is too cold,
or why am I yelling because I have lost my keys? It's then I look at
my calendar and realize, Oh, that's what this is.

SS: Does Dr. Reiss admonish you for not taking them?

MK: Yes, he does. I think there is a little part of me that says, "My
body is supposed to go through this." I have actually been working
with this woman who sees menopause as an opportunity. She thinks
that it is a chance in our lives to embrace the maternal. Not just as
mothers, but to look at ourselves as women and totally accept what
that means, and that it is a moment in time when you are changing;
that it is a step forward into the rest of your life. For me right now
with my TV show, *Friends,* ending, it is almost overwhelming.

SS: So there are a couple of things going on.

MK: Yes, and psychologically a part of me may be avoiding the
next step. Deep down maybe I think that if I am no longer going
to be a fertile woman anymore, some sort of punishment must be
involved with this passage. There is a week each month where I
should be locked in a closet until it is over.

SS: Those are awful weeks. But replacing lost hormones with
natural bioidentical ones helps keep your brain sharp.

MK: Well, that is encouraging because I am a writer, and I am
finding that sometimes I have lost words. Suddenly I can't think of
the word for sock.

I had my third child at forty-three, and it was a very difficult
pregnancy. I was extremely hormonal, which was a different experience. With my other children during pregnancy, I never felt better, or more sexual, or more feminine.

SS: What did your doctor say to you?

MK: He said, "Two hundred and fifty years ago you were supposed to be dead at forty-three." And that really struck me how
fortunate I am not only to be alive, but also to be having a baby.
This made it difficult for me, but I dealt with it with a better sense

of humor. The other thing I notice with my new hormonal imbalance is that my eating has changed.

SS: In what way?

MK: I crave the foods that are worst for me. Like chocolates, sugar, carbohydrates. Also, a year ago I became a vegetarian. On the one hand it has been great, but on the other hand it has been very difficult. I eat fish, but no white or red meat. Well, you can't eat fish three times a day, and cheese doesn't work for me, and dairy makes me sleepy, tired, and sluggish; but when I was on a low-carb, high-protein diet, I felt great and had no cravings at all.

SS: What other changes have you noticed?

MK: I get my period every three weeks now. My doctor said it's kind of like the last hurrah. So probably it will all stop in the next couple of years.

My mom went through menopause when she was fifty, and she acted horribly. I remember her celebrating when she stopped getting her period, and then it was all downhill. So that is the model I have. Maybe that is part of why I am resisting hormones.

SS: I think when the time comes you will not be resistant. The relief is so welcome because you get to feel like your old self again. Normal.

MK: As we are talking I am thinking to myself, Why am I putting myself through this? I have to get back on a schedule with my doctor and take these hormones, because when I think back to when I was taking them regularly, I realize I had tools.

I am having a hard time sleeping. I get about four or five hours a night.

SS: Do you think this is because of hormones or stress?

MK: Not necessarily stress. I've just thought this is what happens as we get older; but when I think about it, my husband sleeps.

My doctor said that if I am having a hard time sleeping to take a couple of extra drops of progesterone and twenty minutes later I will feel relaxed and able to fall asleep. So when I think back on when I was doing that, I realize that was one of the greatest gifts he ever gave me.

SS: So there's your answer.

MK: Yes, this is very good motivation for me to go back to what had worked for me last summer. I guess I got off course.

SS: Do you think that all the negative reports you hear in the media have frightened you away?

MK: That may be part of the problem, that my body is supposed to do this and why am I interfering.

My grandmother aged so magnificently. She was the cutest thing in the whole world with the most beautiful, soft wrinkles. I always wanted to touch her face. She was ninety-three when she died. My mother was much younger when she died.

SS: Did your mother work?

MK: Yes, she worked and she lost my father when she was much younger, plus she was a teenager during the Depression, so she had to work to support her family.

SS: On top of that, she probably had no understanding of menopause, so she suffered through it. But that still doesn't make menopausal women easier to live with.

MK: I know, I feel sorry for my husband.

SS: Yes, but you and I are the lucky ones because we are going through this at an age where younger doctors are saying, "Hey, wait a minute, what we've been doing has not been working; women are not having a good quality of life, plus they are getting diseases: heart disease, stroke, diabetes, plus there is the weight gain."

MK: Yes, but we are also living when pharmaceutical companies have an enormous amount of power, and I find that really frightening.

My doctor, who is cutting-edge, gave me a whole bag of homeopathic medicine before I went into the hospital to have my baby with a C-section. He said, "I can't give you this in the hospital, but I want you to take this twenty-four hours before surgery, and this is what I want you to take as soon as the surgery is over. This is what I want you to put on your skin." Then he said, "As soon as you start feeling postpartum, I want you to come in and I will give you progesterone on the spot." He said, "You are not going to believe how good you are going to feel." And he was right . . . it was as if someone had come in and lifted the dark clouds.

SS: That is the power of hormones and taking natural medicine.

MK: Well, Dr. Reiss is very empowering. His way not only appeals to my common sense, it actually excites me to think about stepping forward proudly, embracing the changes rather than fighting them off, and resolving that I am going through menopause and I don't have to suffer because of the quality care I am getting from my doctor and his understanding of natural hormones.

SS: Do you feel any of the shame that is associated with going through menopause?

MK: It's awful. On the one hand I joke about it, but I feel so undesirable and I can't help but think, how could my husband desire this? Some days I feel like a dried-up old lady. So there is an enormous amount of shame and negativity. But my husband is really trying to be understanding, and I love him for that.

I remember someone saying to me that I had the world at my feet: the big job, a great husband, wonderful children. What is the cost? And I thought. The cost is me, personally. I don't take care of myself because I am so busy taking care of everyone and everything else. Between the work, the kids, making the lunches at night, it's exhausting, because I don't want to give anything up. But I am paying the price personally. So my reluctance to take on menopause and deal with it may be an extension of that.

SS: Do you think you're not worth it on a subliminal level?

MK: Probably . . . always thinking of everyone else.

SS: So finding balance seems to be the key. The key to replacing lost hormones, along with a host of other things, is that it keeps your brain functioning as though you are in your prime. That's very important because now it is coupled with wisdom and perspective. I would think as a writer that would be vitally important to you.

MK: I have never connected that with hormone loss. That alone does make it appealing. I love the new medicine, my doctor gave me a twenty-four-hour urine test, where you collect it hour by hour. He was able to see everything going on in my system—antioxidants, free radicals, health of my heart; he even figured that I didn't have enough salt in my diet.

SS: Yes, this is the new medicine.

MK: I have always shied away from chemicals and synthetics, and somehow hormones were caught up in that. But this new way, with natural bioidentical hormones, is appealing. It helps me to understand that not only would I benefit from replacement, but that I deserve to have quality cutting-edge information and treatment. This helps me into this next passage with new enthusiasm. Thank you.

SS: Good luck, and thank you.

Perks of aging: "I no longer have patience for people who don't like me."

—My friend Susie Weinthal, age 69

7

DR. UZZI REISS, M.D., OB/GYN:
NATURAL HORMONE BALANCE

Dr. Reiss sees six thousand women a year, most of whom come to him suffering from hormonal imbalance. They need help, and he gives them relief. Dr. Reiss is a passionate and fascinating doctor who has demystified the confusing issues surrounding this time of life. He is unique in that as a gynecologist he has researched and learned about the complexities of the hormonal system, which generally is not the specialty of gynecologists. He has been giving women natural hormones for over twenty years. His approach is learned and refreshing because he has stepped outside of the pharmaceutical common course of synthetic hormones, and as a result, women are flocking to him. He recognizes the need for women to understand their hormonal lives. The important phrase here is "natural bioidentical hormones"; Dr. Reiss is a proponent of them, and thousands of women love what he has done for them.

SS: Thank you for speaking with me, Dr. Reiss, I've heard a lot about you.

UR: All good, I hope.

SS: Absolutely. I want to talk about natural hormones. I'm in my middle fifties, and as a woman, I have been programmed all my life to think that this is the beginning of the end and that it's all downhill from here. But I have to say this passage for me is the best I have ever felt, the healthiest I have ever been, the happiest I've ever experienced, and the most fulfilled. Couple all of this with the beginnings of wisdom and perspective, and life is good. I believe the reason I am enjoying such superb quality of life is that I take natural bioidentical hormones and they are balanced.

UR: I agree, replacing bioidentical hormones gives back your quality of life. As a physician, it is my job to understand the side effects, the benefits, and how you can individualize hormone therapy for each particular person. I think the key to all of it is individualization, because women are so different. If we take a thousand women who are twenty years old who say they feel great and are mentally clear, with good energy, perfect weight, great memory, great sex drive, and clear skin, and then you measure their hormones, and for example let's say these women are in the third day of their cycle—you will see thousands of different variations. The goal is for women to achieve the perfect combination for themselves.

SS: Help me to understand . . . how do you determine how much estrogen and how much progesterone?

UR: First I need to find the expression of the hormone inside the cell. We really don't have a direct tool to look inside the cell, so I use a blood test as an indirect tool to tell me if the levels are too high or too low.

Let me tell you how I work. There are three types of women. One is Twiggy.

SS: Twiggy? Skinny, tall, little breasts . . .

UR: Right. Tall, thin, barely any breasts, and barely any muscle. Twiggy never had acne, and you would have to take a microscope to see hair on her body. The Twiggy type is typically very low in both estrogen and testosterone and generally has relatively good human growth hormones because she is tall.

Now let's take someone else who is five feet one, D-size breasts, has no hair over her body, is not very athletic, and does not have strong muscles; this woman has extremely high estrogen, and low testosterone.

SS: This is the curvy body?

UR: Right, this woman has about six- to sevenfold more estrogen than Twiggy. Estrogen has indeed built her breasts and has given her a happy mentality. I don't want to generalize, but women of this type are happier and less complex, and it seems that their approach to sexuality is much simpler.

Then we have the intermediate group, what I call the athlete. If you notice, most women athletes have small breasts. Not because they have low estrogen, but because they have high testosterone. You can't be an athlete and have low testosterone, nor can you be a dancer and have low testosterone, because you wouldn't have the spatial coordination and balance that testosterone gives you. Also (and I'm generalizing) athletes have nice muscles.

You see, hormone is a language, and each hormone has its own language. Hormones do specific things that they have been doing for the last billion years of evolution. A hormone is not only a number, it's also an expression of specific mentality, specific attitudes.

Let's take a simple example: A lady comes to me and says that lately she is bleeding less during her period, her vagina is dry, and her breasts are droopy. The only thing it can be is that she is making less estrogen. Estrogen builds up the lining in the uterus. When there is less estrogen, there is less lining and thus less of a period. When I give her estrogen, it fills the breast, so now the breasts are less droopy. Estrogen gives women vaginal lubrication, so when I give her estrogen the vagina becomes less dry.

We know that women have fluctuations in their estrogen during their normal cycle. A woman tends to have lower estrogen before her period than the week after because her body wants to prepare the lining of the uterus for implantation, so it shoots up the estrogen levels. If a woman comes to me and says she has been feeling good, but in the last two years she feels good only the week after she finishes her period, then I have my answer. This is the week the body makes more estrogen.

SS: So what do you do for her at this point?

UR: I start to ask specific questions. Estrogen is vitally important because it gives women their great mind; estrogen makes women happy. We have to think of what women were supposed to do fifty thousand years ago. Women's bodies are adjusted not to the life we have today, but to life fifty thousand years ago. At that time women were the center and had all the power. They were responsible for feeding everyone and keeping everyone together and happy. Women with normal estrogen are happy and outgoing, they want to teach, they want to give, they also need a lot of good deep sleep—they don't have much time left in each day because they are so busy giving of themselves.

SS: And balanced estrogen ensures a good night's sleep.

UR: Correct. That's why when a woman starts losing estrogen she has interrupted sleep.

SS: Are estrogen-dominant women happier in general than a testosterone woman?

UR: In a certain way, yes. For example, have you met a lot of models?

SS: Yes.

UR: They are tall, thin, and usually sort of subtly depressed. I ask these same women how they were feeling when they were pregnant and they usually say it was the happiest they ever felt.

This goes back to the patient's individual hormonal history, which I factor in when I design a hormonal treatment plan for that woman. I treat women with hormones from age fourteen to the age of ninety. Hormone therapy is considered the domain of menopausal women, but it applies to every age. Many women never reach their hormonal balance, which is sad because it is so easy to feel great when you find balance.

I see so many women every year. When a woman comes to see me before her period (when her estrogen is low), she usually dresses more conservatively (this is especially so with menopausal women—they dress darker and are less body conscious). The week after she is finished with her period she is happy, dresses more colorfully, is more body conscious, and cares more about her body.

When a woman comes to my office and tells me she doesn't feel right in her body anymore, I think about her with the history of hormones in mind. I usually know what is wrong before she tells me by her body shape, size, and the way she describes how she is feeling. Usually her estrogen is low. I have done this for twenty years, and I know I can't be right all the time, but the majority of the time it is the correct assessment.

Now, here is another situation where hormones are dynamic. If after you finish writing this book I send you and your husband to Tahiti for a month, and all you do is light exercise, and rest on the beach all day long, your estrogen requirements will go down by 30 percent. Last time I took my wife to Hawaii her estrogen dropped 30 to 40 percent. On the other hand, if you decide to train for a marathon, your body will consume more estrogen and you will have to increase it. That's why a "one pill fits all" as in synthetic so-called hormones can't work. Every day your hormone requirements change. When a woman is stressed, she decreases a substance in her body called cyclic AMP. It is a messenger that goes from the brain of the cell to the outskirts of the cell to get the information the hormones give to it. This messenger barely works when you are stressed.

SS: So it is up to the woman to evaluate her stress levels to know when she needs to call her doctor and get reevaluated.

UR: Most of the time I teach women how to increase and decrease the amount of hormones they use based upon how they feel and their stress levels. A few of these cases are more complex because of the degree of the problem and the fact that patients respond differently to the hormone treatment. These women require constant guidance in the initial stages of their treatment. For instance, I have a patient who came to me after having had a hysterectomy nine months ago. She has been constantly suicidal because her hormones have been so out of balance. But now, after three weeks of treating her with various doses of hormones, she is nearly a normal person.

SS: Wow! That's incredible. I know so many women who have had hysterectomies who are miserable and at times suicidal. What did you do for her?

UR: Basically, I kept adjusting and tracking the doses of estrogen and progesterone.

I think it's very important to understand that we are living in an era with the biggest assault on womanhood in history. Everyday stress takes away a woman's estrogen, and with it her sensuality, her sexuality, her smartness, her beauty, her serenity, her sleep, her memory, her passion, and her sensitivity. The stress of today's life is assaulting her estrogen, but women have become frightened of hormones because reports come out that say they are going to kill you or give you cancer.

SS: Well, what are they supposed to think when so many negative reports are put out by the media?

UR: Yes, and this information is flawed. These reports, which are always about synthetic hormones and not natural bioidentical hormones, are constantly being thrust in women's faces. These flawed studies are frightening women away from estrogen. Every day I see women who are nearly falling apart because their estrogen has been taken away from them either because their body has stopped making it or they have read these reports and stopped taking it on their own.

They have no choice but to turn to the alternatives: a sleeping pill to sleep, antianxiety pills to relax, antidepressant pills to take away their depression, Ritalin to make their memory a little better . . . And what you get is a pharmaceutical product that loses humanity.

SS: So many of the women I have talked with regarding this subject repeat the same thing: "I feel dead inside."

UR: Yes, this form of treatment takes the soul out of them. It takes away what I call the vibration of living.

Recently there was another study by the Women's Health Initiative done on Provera, a chemicalized progesterone. Provera is known to be destructive to the heart. It can close the coronary arteries, enhance the growth of arterial plaque, and make it unstable so there will be more heart attacks. There is existing literature on this drug. It is known to leech calcium from bone, and it is also known to aggressively increase breast cancer; what they haven't told you yet is that Provera is totally destructive to the brain, because Provera is like MSG. A bad MSG. Now that you know what this drug does, you understand why the study that used this drug resulted in such a bad outcome. It is not favorable to the brain. It overuses the brain, then crushes the cells.

The second drug used in this study was Premarin, an extract from the urine of pregnant mares (female horses). In other words, this is a substance that nature never intended for the bodies of human females. If we said that estrogen was the base of your mind, your mood, and your memory, then I ask you: is there anything similar between a woman and a pregnant mare? Here we have two billion years of general evolution and two million years of human evolution, and we are giving women two pharmaceutically designed hormones totally different from the hormones a woman makes in her own body.

SS: Why doesn't the medical community understand this? Why are we not giving women hormones that are an exact replica?

UR: Because natural bioidentical hormones cannot be patented. No one wants to spend money on studies of a hormone that can be copied by other companies. Instead, synthetic hormones can be patented and advertised, and no one can copy them.

Here is an example: Let's say papaya is expensive and the sellers need to put DDT in it so it will preserve itself and have a longer shelf life and also more people will be able to afford it. Then a report comes out that papaya with DDT is shown to increase breast cancer. What would be your journalistic conclusion? That papaya increases breast cancer? No. DDT increases breast cancer!

What most people don't realize is that the scientific technology for creating bioidentical hormones [hormones identical to those in our bodies] has been around for fifty years. But instead they decided to use Premarin because horses have huge bladders, and they can feed them hay, which is really inexpensive, keep them in small stalls, catheterize their bladders, and give them tranquilizers to keep them calm, so they can easily make tons of estrogen. So it's about business. But the estrogen from horses' urine is not an exact replica of what we make in our bodies. Only bioidentical HRT, synthesized in a lab, made from plant extracts, exactly replicates what our own bodies make.

The study on Premarin began fifty years ago. They started giving natural hormones to women who were menopausal. Without a doubt, thousands of studies on women from different places around the world showed the following: 50 percent decrease in Alzheimer's disease, 50 percent decrease in heart attacks, 50 percent decrease in bone loss, 50 percent decrease in blindness, and now we know 50 percent decrease in colon cancer.

With Premarin they give estrogen alone, but in the physiology of the body, estrogen always goes with progesterone. Normal physiology is required amounts of estrogen every day of the month, and progesterone on days one through fourteen. If estrogen goes up, then progesterone goes up; if estrogen goes down, then progesterone goes down. But in giving estrogen alone, women started to develop mild forms of uterine cancer. There was no balance and this is the connection that made all this mania about estrogen and uterine cancer. In addition, because Premarin is like a foreign substance to the human body, the body reacts by increasing the inflammation process. If this reaction is sustained for five to fifteen years because the foreign substance is continuously introduced to the body, it will increase the incidence of heart disease and Alzheimer's, thereby negating the original benefit.

SS: Meaning that our bodies make estrogen and progesterone and that to eliminate one of these important hormones creates imbalance, and imbalance—

UR: Creates disease. Because it was not estrogen that caused the cancer, it was the lack of progesterone. For instance, if I removed your eyes and then asked you to drive a car, you would have an accident because I took away your vision. It's the same thing. The two hormones work in concert with each other.

Now when pharmaceutical companies realized that the two hormones were important, they had to find a way to patent them. So they decided to change them pharmaceutically, and that is how synthetic hormones became the common treatment.

The way I work is, I teach women how to have control over the natural hormones they take. The modern woman is a new experiment; she is the woman who is pregnant only one or two times in her life, and she is working outside the home. These women are not healthier; they have more disease. At the beginning of the century, there was no endometriosis, there were not a lot of fibroids and not a lot of the diseases we have today.

SS: Don't you think this might be environmental?

UR: Definitely. Our unhealthful environment makes us more prone to illness and also "confuses" the natural function of our hormones. Processed foods and the materials they are packaged in are full of artificial hormones that compete with and therefore confuse women's natural hormonal balance. This, plus the enormous tasks placed on the shoulders of women in our society, makes it nearly impossible for modern women to achieve many things that are dearest to them.

I have a sentence I often say: Pregnancy is not the beginning of the extension of the family, it is the beginning of the extinction of the family.

SS: What do you mean?

UR: It's because women focus all their attention on their children and stop thinking about themselves and their relationship with their husbands. I advise every woman before she does anything when she gets up in the morning, to think about what she is going to do for herself today and what she is going to do for her partner to make their relationship grow and get better. So many women tell me that they are unable to have sex with their husbands because of the kids. By the time she puts the kids to bed, she usually falls asleep with them, then wakes up at two in the morning and her husband is already asleep, then the kids come into the bed in the morning. Women today need to reprioritize their lives.

SS: Maybe they use this as an excuse to avoid sex, and maybe that's because they are off hormonally, perhaps low testosterone.

UR: Low testosterone is not always the case. For instance, a woman athlete has high testosterone all her life. The problem is that when you take away a woman's estrogen she can't do anything with her testosterone. Testosterone by itself just makes her aggressive. When a woman is going through menopause, or is just before her period, her estrogen starts to go down: Once the estrogen goes down, the testosterone goes way up. So she goes from being serene, loving, open, and sexual to being moody, depressed, and uninterested in going outside and enjoying herself. Instead she gets mean, bitchy, upset, and short-tempered.

I saw a woman on TV who wrote a book about menopause, and I heard her say that menopause has healing power . . . she said, "I felt strong and I finally had the guts to throw him out." I say no, you lost your estrogen. Estrogen is the hormone that gives women that wonderful balance between strength, clear thinking, and patience. It makes them wise and tolerant. On the other hand, when estrogen levels sink during menopause, a woman's body releases more testosterone, which causes women to be aggressive but without that soft, clear-thinking, patient component to balance the aggression. This is the reason that many women are perceived as overly emotional during menopause. But it doesn't have to be this way. There must always be a balance between estrogen and testosterone levels.

SS: What about women who are estrogen dominant? Is that a good thing?

UR: Actually, very few women are estrogen dominant. Those who are dominant are happy and clear, but they usually have a tremendous amount of water retention, bloating, and breast tenderness and extremely heavy periods, because estrogen builds a lot of lining. In reality this woman is not estrogen dominant, she simply lacks progesterone. In menopause, when this woman starts losing her estrogen, she will get depressed and foggy, will not sleep well, and will tend to turn inward.

SS: What are the health ramifications of a woman who is estrogen dominant?

UR: She may have a slightly higher incidence of endometriosis, fibroids, and cystic breasts. But it is not from estrogen, it is from lack of progesterone. Once I give these women progesterone, I often find that now their estrogen is blocked, and it is here I discover that they are also estrogen deficient. Then I have to add a little more estrogen to find balance.

SS: Every woman's needs are different.

UR: Yes, and it takes time to find the right balance for each woman. We were all created perfect. The great thing about bioidentical hormones is that we can always find a match for your individual optimal requirements. The beauty of bioidentical hormones is that they talk to you: if you give too much, you have side effects; the same goes for testosterone, DHEA, HGH, thyroid, and the adrenal hormones. All of them are a beautiful orchestra, and it is possible to teach every woman to find balance by herself. They learn when to take a little more and when to take a little less.

SS: And when is that?

UR: It depends. At any age, hormones in the body are fluctuating. So let's take estrogen (and every woman should check with her doctor before doing this): You wake up in the morning and your thinking is a little foggy or uninspired, and you don't feel motivated, then you would take a little more of the estrogen cream. If, however, you wake up in the morning and you are a little uptight, and your breasts are tender, take minimally less. Very few women come to me and say they don't get it. The amazing thing is that we are now in an era of multiple hormonal deficiencies. It is not just estrogen; it can be thyroid or adrenal. (We could talk forever about the adrenal glands.) When a woman comes in the first time, I can't be sure which hormone deficiency is dominant, so I start her on the hormones I feel are the most needed, based upon her history and the results of her blood tests. But with time, some of the hormonal deficiencies that I believed were dominant reveal themselves to be *reactions* to the deficiencies of other hormones. From this point on, the course of treatment will focus on the "true" deficiencies.

SS: Which do you start with, progesterone or estrogen?

UR: It depends upon the situation. Recently I saw through blood work that a patient of mine was in menopause. She complained of breast tenderness and water retention. I could see through lab work that she still had some estrogen, but not the optimal amount; but she has it all the time, so we call it unopposed. This woman had certain signs of too much estrogen, but general signs of not enough—for instance, her vagina is dry, her mind is foggy, and she cannot sleep. With someone like this, I first prescribe progesterone. Progesterone is a very complex hormone, because only very young women respond to it in the way the textbooks say. Ninety-five percent of the time when you give progesterone to a young woman, she responds to it, she relaxes and calms down. But up to 50 percent of women in menopause who haven't been exposed to progesterone for a few years can react to it as if it were a toxic drug, because it drops the estrogen levels. They feel depressed, or it gives them panic attacks.

Balancing hormones is a work of art, but you can teach women how to do it. I know this because I get letters from my female patients all over the country who have taught themselves. The biggest problem I run into is that every compounding pharmacy is different, and when I write hormone prescriptions (Rx) in one pharmacy, but in another pharmacy it has another quantity, that makes it more difficult.

SS: Why isn't there any standardization?

UR: Because bioidentical hormones are not profitable, so no one is interested in funding the studies.

SS: Well, how does one know which one is a good compounding pharmacy?

UR: If a woman has a favorite pharmacy, or she comes to me from out of town and there is only one in her vicinity, I tell her that the amount I am giving her generally works, but if she is not getting the desired relief, I suggest she get her hormones from a compounding pharmacy that I work with through mail order, where I know she will get better absorption.*

SS: Yes, but isn't there the danger, especially with hormones, of thinking, If a little is good, then a lot will be much better?

---

* See the Resources for a list of compounding pharmacies.

UR: Well, if that were the case, why would diabetics (even children) be allowed to control themselves with insulin? We know that if you let people control themselves, the control is ten times better than having a doctor from remote deciding every month what they can use.

I tell women how to use their hormones, I prescribe the initial dose, then two to three months into the program they come back to my office so I can track their levels. Then I adjust and explain how to control the dose by paying attention to how they are feeling.

SS: What about taking natural hormones when you have breast cancer?

UR: Do you know that one of the oldest descriptions of reasons for breast cancer is lack of DHEA? This is one of the theories that has stood the test of time. Several studies have associated higher levels of DHEA in the body with a lowered incidence of cancer.

SS: But what about those of us who took birth control pills in the 1960s and 1970s? Do you think there is any connection between birth control pills and breast cancer? I am asking only because there is such a high incidence of breast cancer with women of my age group.

UR: You are talking about the most aggressively strong estrogen ever created. When you take estrogen that is that strong, your brain stops making your own estrogen. This is the essence of how it works. When you use natural estrogen, your brain continues to produce it because your body is still fluctuating. Yet they did a study of women on birth control pills and found there was no increase of breast cancer in this group.

SS: What do you think about that?

UR: I think this is another piece of information indicating a Twiggy type: I cannot say that she will never get breast cancer and that someone with large breasts will, even though the estrogen differences between the two women is around sixfold, and in pregnancy it is about tenfold.

We do not know exactly why women get breast cancer, but it doesn't seem to appear that one of the reasons is birth control pills. The literature is mounted with data, but there is never clear scientific evidence that estrogen increases breast cancer. It appears to me that it is the lack of progesterone, or a lack of balance between the two.

Recently, the Nurses' Health Study II, conducted at the Harvard School of Public Health, published its findings regarding folic acid and breast cancer. The study compared women with the lowest folic acid levels to women with the highest folic acid levels. Women with the highest folic acid levels had 89 percent less chance of breast cancer than women with low folic acid levels. Now "they" say folic acid "may make a difference," but we already know this about folic acid. The scientific reason is that folic acid inhibits the production of 4-hydroxyestrone, an aggressive type of estrogen that can mutate DNA and start the cancer process. In other words, folic acid helps in the prevention of breast cancer.

The women I see are not forced to come to me; they come from all over the world wanting cutting-edge information. They want to combine everything—mind, nutrients, and hormones—and work toward building a protective modality toward everything in their bodies.

SS: It's clear that there are changes in the wind, but it is very hard for women to find a doctor like you. Many gynecologists are prescribing hormones, and it is not their specialty. I am finding in my research that a standard approach for many gynecologists is to give a complaining menopausal woman antidepressants like Paxil or Prozac.

UR: Yes, and that will destroy their sex lives totally. The antidepressant takes away their anxiety resulting from lack of hormones, so they think they feel better and forget that they have a sex drive deficiency. They just feel flat, or as I say, they lose their vibration of living.

You see, women are superior to men from a health aspect: they live longer and survive longer. But for every man who takes an antidepressant, twenty women are taking it; for every man who takes antianxiety medication, twenty women are taking it; for every man who takes a sleeping pill, twenty women are taking it.

SS: Why is that?

UR: It is estrogen . . . too much or too little. That's why finding balance is so important. The problem with doctors giving hormones is that for the most part they don't give hormones, they give drugs. Pharmaceutical companies take hormones and change them, and these changes form side effects.

Bioidentical hormones give such great benefits; you have the wisdom of aging, but balanced hormones allow you to run and fly with it.

I look at many people who are aging who have not addressed their hormonal selves, and they have turned monotonic; their behavior is old, uninspired, they don't want any challenges, they want everything to be repetitious, and they are more cynical. Hormones are the essence of living as long as we don't try to change them. We are not to play God with nature, and we must respect the physiological process. Hormone replacement is a tool to stay in the game.

SS: What is your hope for the future?

UR: That women will have the choices to decide what they want to do hormonally, then learn how to individualize them, and use them continuously to be able to run, grow, dream, hope, learn, and challenge themselves. Yes, women are confused, but confusion is good when they hear an orchestra of different opinions; if women hear just one opinion, that is depressing, like a black cloud or a tunnel without an end or light. I think the light is coming and more women are hearing about it.

SS: Thank you so much.

these really
ARE THE
sexy years!

Signs of menopause: You're on so much estrogen that you take your Brownie troop on a field trip to Chippendale's.

8
SEX

It seems unfair that finally we've reached a time in our lives when we have the time for sex but not the inclination. All those years when our heads were so cluttered with lists and the needs of the children: the dance lessons, the soccer practice, Little League games, cupcakes for the class on school birthdays, the parent-teacher meetings . . . then there were the business activities and the dinner parties, getting it right and all that that entails. Sex was always something that your husband was just going to have to wait for, because how can you be thinking about quality orgasms when you have so much to do and so little time? Wasn't getting into bed at night the first time in the day when you were able to think for yourself about what needed to be done, and now *he* wants to have sex? Did you do it because he needed it, with a "let's just get it over with" attitude so he could go to sleep so you could *finally have some time for yourself?*

Okay, you've done your job now. You've done it well. The kids have kids of their own. There are no more lessons or sports activities, the business dinners are not so important anymore. You have more time to spend with your husband. It's great, you can get dressed up, go out, enjoy stimulating, mature conversation, have a great dinner that someone else prepares, have a few drinks, go home, and make wild and crazy love. Is that what is happening? If not, let me tell you, it can and should be. This is the greatest time of your life. But here's the problem: If you are "not in the mood," or if there just isn't any desire, it's because you have zeroed out hormonally. That means testosterone, too. Yes, we women have testosterone. When we stop making this hormone along with estrogen and progesterone, it's like the gas in your car running out. Without the gas, the car won't go; it doesn't matter if you push it, jump-start it, or roll it down a hill, it needs gas to operate. That's how it works with us.

Now you may feel, So what, I don't care if I have sex anymore. . . . Believe me, it's only because you have forgotten how great it can be. It also might be that your partner has been less than charismatic in the romance department. It does take two. Or it might be that you have been having gratuitous sex for so long and acting like nothing more than a receptacle all these years so that you could "get it over with." Whatever bad habits have been established, you have the power and the information to change these habits—you just need the will to do so.

The first thing you have to do is deal with your hormones. You know how important it is to do so from reading the last chapters. Have your blood work tracked to see what your levels are relative to progesterone, estrogen, DHEA, and testosterone, especially the free testosterone levels. Free testosterone determines your sexual vigor (more about testosterone and free testosterone in the next chapter). Now here's the tricky part. Very few doctors understand what to do with these levels. If there isn't a good endocrinologist in your area whose specialty is natural bioidentical hormones, insist that your doctor lead you to the right professional. This might take some work, but it is so worth it. You need to figure out which hormones you are lacking, because when you are able to replenish the ones you are missing and get your hormonal system in balance, you will notice a dramatic change in how you feel about sex. You will actually want it! I promise you when you get this figured out, you're going to be thinking of ways to drag your guy into the bedroom.

Balancing your hormones will not only make you want and enjoy sex more, it will also help keep your marriage intact. Have

you noticed how many men leave their wives at middle age? Why
is that? You're looking good, you're in good shape, the two of you
are best friends. Why would he ever leave you? Remember, men
also experience loss of hormones. Their testosterone levels are
diminishing at the same time you are losing yours. Shouldn't that
put you on an equal path? The answer is no. Never underestimate
a man's need to be virile. Your husband's midlife is just as discon-
certing to him as yours is to you. He is losing his ability to have an
erection anytime he wants. Before, all he had to do was think
about it, and bingo! There it is in all its mighty glory . . . erect and
tall, ready for action. But now, maybe it doesn't last as long, and
it's not as mighty as it once was, and sometimes it doesn't want to
salute at all. You aren't the only one who should be getting your
hormones checked out. It's also time for him to get to the endocrinologist and have his DHEA and testosterone levels checked.
That's all it takes for him—the endocrinologist can prescribe a
dosage of hormones tailored exactly to what he requires once he's
checked his levels.

I'll tell you more about men and andropause (male menopause)
and what they are going through in part 4, where you can find out
exactly what your husband is experiencing as he gets older, physically, mentally, and sexually, and how balancing his hormones can
take care of these challenges. What he has lost in the aging process
can be restored that easily, although most men are too embarrassed
to try to find out what is wrong. It's not their fault; it's just how
our society has approached raising men. We have been telling our
sons "not to cry" and "act like a man," telling them what men do
and don't do, leaning on them to handle all those things that are
not in our realm. So our men have assumed the mantle because
that is what is expected of them.

Suddenly at middle age, they're not going to be able to reveal
lack of vitality or something as vulnerable as sexual dysfunction.
But I tell you again—we are going to live almost twice as long as
our grandparents, and we have to deal with the second half differently. The scary part is that most men (did you hear me), *most*

men, think the problem is you, that you don't turn him on any-more. And let's face it, you probably haven't been a real pistol in that area. So what do they do? To prove that they still have "lead in their pencils," they go out and find themselves the new, improved, younger version of you. That's why you see so many old guys with young wives and new babies. It is terribly sad for the families left behind. The children you raised together feel rejected, that they're no longer the "real" family, that the new babies in their father's life are the preferred ones. It's a syndrome that is hap-pening all around us, and it's avoidable if you can understand the part you are playing in this scenario.

Relationships require "work" that never stops as long as you are together. You must understand that all those nights when you "weren't in the mood," or went through the motions without putting any effort into the act, spelled the beginning of the end. Time after time of having thoughtless sex, of feelingless, emotion-less sex, adds up. At some point both of you stop trying. Then it is reduced to an occasional "wham bam, thank you, ma'am." At some point he's going to look elsewhere, even if he doesn't want to. There will be some new "babe" in the office who sees him as her ticket to life. After all, your husband has spent a lifetime building his business or perfecting his job so that he's now well paid and respected. Young girls find that very attractive. Many young girls don't want to go through the rough times with a guy their age. They'd like to start at the point of success. They want to move into a big house without all the trials and tribulations. They also might be looking for someone more mature. Frankly, who could blame them?

I tell you, get your hormones together and then get to work. This is for you. Stop just "lying there." Get involved. Lose weight, buy some great underwear; plan some weekends at your favorite places. Pick out places conducive to lying around having great sex. Do the things to him that you know he loves, and then do them *really well.* He will love it. *Love it!* All men love to be taken care of sexually. Don't fake that you are enjoying yourself—get into it and you'll find that you will love it, too. After all, this is your man; this is the guy you've chosen to spend your life with; this is the father of your children. He's been with you through all of it. Think about those things while you are pleasing him. You will start to feel such deep love for him that giving him this pleasure will become something you both look forward to doing. If you feel awkward and don't know if you are using the right technique, and many of us don't, rent a video or watch those kinds of movies on cable. You can learn from watching them. Once you become comfortable and look forward to this being a regular part of sex for the two of you, be sure to have him show you exactly what he wants.

The wrong technique can be a turnoff. Every man is different. Relearn what your guy likes. You used to know how to excite him, and believe me, you will get very turned on when you know you are in control because you are giving him the most intense pleasure. When he is so aroused you can feel that he is ready to explode, it is very exciting for you. It is this intensity that makes you want to do it again and again. When sex becomes like this, no one and nothing can come between the two of you.

Believe me, a man who is getting great sex at home, and I mean horny, involved sex, is not going to be attracted to anyone outside of you. No middle-aged man walks around saying, "Boy, would I love to have a few new babies in my life. Yes, sir, I really want to get back into diapers, nursery school, baby-sitters, PTA, and teacher conferences." The reason these middle-aged men are having babies is that it's part of the deal of getting all this new and horny sex. Don't allow your relationship to digress anywhere near to this state. Take charge of your life now. Surprise him. Maybe the first time it will be awkward, but tell him why you are interested in changing your sex life. Try to really talk about the fact that this part of your life has been ignored, but that you want to change things. The discomfort will dissipate quickly.

Tell him you love him and that it's his time now. Tell him that you're sorry you've spent so many years making him last in line in the family. Tell him that you want a different kind of marriage now. This is a new passage. Make sex dates. You can go out for a nice dinner at your favorite romantic restaurant, come home, fill the bathtub, and get in with him. Have fun, laugh, wash his back, and ask him to wash yours. It will work. But don't be discouraged if he doesn't respond the way you want him to the first, second, or third time. This will be new to him, and you have trained him all these years that sex was last on your list of favorite activities. Then make love to him as though today were the last day you would ever be together in your lives. Imagine that. If you knew this was the last time, how would you act?

Now, I say this: If you don't want to do this, if it's too much effort, if the idea of it is totally unappealing, then you have to examine what you really want. If it's not worth it to put this much effort into rejuvenating your relationship, then maybe this relationship is not what you want.

On the other hand, if this is where you want to go in your relationship—if what you want is to love and be loved, to feel secure and trusting, to have an easy communication, respect, openness, and great sex—then "give it a go," as they say in England.

Keep in mind that part of the deal in pleasing your partner in ways he's never or rarely experienced is that you are part of the equation. This isn't all about him. You have to tell him what it is sexually that you've wanted in your relationship together. Anyone who has gone to certain religious schools (I attended Catholic) was groomed in a way that led to a lot of sexual hang-ups. The word was that sex and physical intimacy were to be saved for marriage only, so all the natural thoughts you had about sex in your teen years were accompanied by enormous guilt. It was a sin even to think of it, let alone "do it." My religious upbringing required that you confess your "sins" every Saturday, and that would entail the humiliating aspect of explaining your "impure thoughts," or worse, confessing that you allowed a body part to be touched. It doesn't take long before every "impure thought" makes you sick with guilt and you will do just about anything to talk yourself out of finding any kind of enjoyment in any sexual act. Then voilà, you get married and you're supposed to be some kind of little sex pistol in bed. I was afraid even to open my eyes. I became pregnant in my teen years, having had sex only one time. It wasn't really even sex as I have come to know it. It doesn't matter, because the greatest joy and achievement of my life was bringing my son, Bruce, into this world. But my point is, how do you go from one extreme to another without having some residual hang-ups?

So now what's in it for you? We're talking sexually. What do you want? First of all, when your head is focused and "there," it doesn't matter what the two of you do together as long as you are both enjoying yourself. But your involvement has to be real. If you have been faking enjoyment all these years, you can no longer do so. What's the point? The object at this age is to realize that anything the two of you want to do together is good and beautiful. You have chosen to spend your entire lives together. You know how to please him outside of the usual positions; you know how to add the element of surprise and extra pleasure. But what about you? The missionary position can be great, but has he learned about pleasing you outside of the usual things you have been doing all these years?

Most women are too embarrassed to teach their mates exactly what to do. He has to be shown. Our bodies are mysteries to men in so many ways. There are caverns and folds, layer upon layer of erotic possibilities. Most women don't want to be "traffic cops," so they feel reluctant to tell their partner where to go and what to do; but good sex requires that you physically show him what you like. Once he knows what you love, sex will be unbelievably exciting to both of you. A man can't ever understand our bodies in the way we do. They have a different physical makeup, and as we need them to teach us, without embarrassment, what feels good to their bodies, we also need to teach them how to touch us, where to touch us, and with what intensity.

It takes time and willingness for both of you to learn what works for you. The good news is that this is one place where men have all the patience in the world. They want us to have great orgasms. It is much more intense and enjoyable for men when we are as turned on as they are—or even more so! He can't rely upon knowledge from other women he has been with because we all have different likes and dislikes. But don't rely solely upon him doing all the work. Looking and watching each other during sex also adds to the erotic quality of the experience. It is uncomfortable at first if you have been used to keeping your eyes closed (as I did in my early years), but it is one of those things that makes sex "hornier." If talking to your mate about sex is too awkward, try going to a sex therapist.

Why not do these things? We're talking about getting the most out of life and enjoying the freedom and maturity that are the inherent gifts of coming to this age. What are you waiting for? You've earned the right to have all the pleasure your body can experience. You've already been the good mother, the perfect housewife, and gone to the top in your career. There is nothing left to prove. From this point on, anything you accomplish is something you do for yourself, not for outside approval. Everyone around you is already impressed with you as a person. You've done it well. But this is for you. Have you ever noticed that some women have a certain confidence about them, as if they have validation from within? These are the women who have already figured this out. They aren't worried that their husbands or partners will stray because they know they are both getting everything they want at home. It's beyond sex; it's comfort, security, love, laughter, intelligent conversation, shared ideas, family, grandchildren, great meals, and beautiful homes. Put all of this together and the two of you will be having such a great time as a couple that each of you becomes all the other needs. Anything and anyone from the outside is simply frosting.

This is all yours to live and own, but it requires a commitment and a willingness to shift your thinking. You've got to commit to this the same way you would commit to a weight loss program. I always ask my "Somersizers" to make a "shift in your thinking," meaning that it is time to understand that your old patterns of behavior are no longer serving you well. In other words, they're not working, and the only thing you can do to reverse the situation and put it back on track is decide to change. Change requires commitment. "Today I will begin the rest of my life anew." It's truly as simple as that. Decide that you want to change and then do whatever work is necessary to make it happen.

You are in complete and total charge of your life and happiness, and that includes your sexual happiness. Now that you know how important hormones are and what role they play in sexuality, you have no excuse for not getting your blood work done to find out what hormones are depleted. If you don't make it happen, then you have to accept your unhappiness as something you have created. To put the blame on another is useless and futile. You have to take responsibility for your sexual fulfillment. If you start every sentence with "He always . . ." or "He never . . ." or "He won't . . . ," then you are looking for excuses to fail. Who wins in that scenario? Believe me, and as my friend Barry always says: "The only person who knows what you want out of life is you, and no one will be sorrier than you if you don't get it. You've got to choose to fight for what you want, no matter how difficult or insurmountable it appears to be." So go out and get your hormones evaluated. Talk to your husband about your sexual needs. Work on being fun and flirty with him. Fight for your happiness. It's a noble fight. Wouldn't the world be a wonderful place if everyone in it were happy? Idealistic? Yes, but why not? It's up to each and every one of us to make our lives the best they can be. There is no better time and no better age than right now. You finally have all the tools. You have the wisdom. You have perspective. Now go get it!

Old is when . . . your partner says,
"Let's go upstairs and make love," and you
answer, "Pick one, I can't do both."

9

TESTOSTERONE:
SEX IN A CAPSULE

Recently the media has been focusing on the decreased sex drive in women. Without professing any understanding of the role balanced hormones play in our sex drive, the television reports are telling those of us of a certain age to get testosterone cream from our gynecologists. Without hesitation our doctors are prescribing this magic potion. Hooray! Finally, a solution! But hold on, not so fast. Doesn't it sound too good to be true? Could it really be that easy? It's not quite that simple, though testosterone cream does indeed stir things up and make you feel kind of "wiggly" down there.

How can applying testosterone as a cream or taking it in pill form help restore a flagging libido? As you know, testosterone is the hormone that affects sexual desire, and there must be a balanced ratio in our bodies among amounts of estrogen, progesterone, and testosterone. Testosterone is considered mostly the male hormone because it is responsible for masculine characteristics like facial hair and a deep voice, but it is also present in much smaller amounts in women. Like estrogen, testosterone is produced by the ovaries and adrenal glands and declines gradually throughout a woman's life. Testosterone is so central to a woman's sexual function that no lover and no amount of sexual stimulation can make up for its absence. Low testosterone in women creates widely varying symptoms. Some women never notice the difference, while others are devastated by a sudden or gradual decline in libido, especially those who have had a hysterectomy and both ovaries removed. Testosterone levels decline by about a third in perimenopausal women who have had both ovaries removed. Many doctors are reluctant to prescribe testosterone because it has masculinizing side effects like increased facial hair and a deepening of the voice. It can also cause weight gain and acne. More serious side effects associated with higher doses include an increase in cholesterol levels and the risk of liver and heart disease. That is why, if you feel taking testosterone will help your sex drive, it is essential that you be under the care of a good endocrinologist (or a doctor who has made natural bioidentical hormone replacement his or her specialty) who will give you only the amount your body needs through blood testing.

Before a doctor prescribes testosterone, he or she should test your blood levels for two values: total testosterone and free testosterone.

> **The normal range of total testosterone in a premenopausal woman is typically between 10 and 55 ng/dL.**
>
> **A postmenopausal woman's normal levels are 7 to 40 ng/dL.**
>
> **A woman with little muscle and body hair might have a level of 20 to 40 ng/dL.**
>
> **A more muscular and hairy woman will probably have levels of 75 to 100 ng/dL.**

The availability of testosterone in the body is governed directly by the presence of the sex hormone–binding globulin (SHBG). It is also governed indirectly by estrogen. A naturally high estrogen level, or estrogen replacement, translates to an increase in SHBG. That means more testosterone is bound up and the actual level of available (free) testosterone is reduced. For this reason, it is important to have your free testosterone levels checked as well. Every woman is different. Indicators say that .06 ng/dL of free testosterone is right in the middle range and more than adequate for a normal, healthy sex drive. But I have no sex drive at all if my free testosterone levels reach .06. You need to be attuned to your body's needs. Even though my levels register in the normal range, my body requires more. It is up to me to inform my doctor how I am feeling so that she can make adjustments.

Dr. Uzzi Reiss says that a good indicator for a starting dose of testosterone is the amount of body hair and musculature. He says to start low if you have comparatively little hair and muscle development, or if you have more than average hair and more ample muscle development but a testosterone level over 40 ng/dL. Have your doctor increase your dosage gradually. There is a direct dosage relationship to benefits and side effects. The more you take, the more the potential benefits; but the more you take, the more potential side effects also. Your body will tell you within two to six weeks if you are taking the right amount.

Too much testosterone can have an effect on your personality. People might think you have become aggressive and pushy. Pay attention to your moods—if you are acting more aggressive than normal, maybe you are taking too much testosterone. Watch your body, too—if your skin becomes unnaturally oily, if you begin to have acne, if you start to grow too much facial hair or lose hair on your head, then you may be taking too much testosterone. Remember, too much or too little of any hormone creates imbalance and wreaks havoc with your system. You will not get hornier if you take too much testosterone—you will feel as wiggly as you did in your prime only when you are in complete balance. Balance is what we are after.

Testosterone comes in gel, cream, drops, inserted pellets, and capsule form. Some women experience adequate day-long benefits after taking testosterone once in the morning. Others may need it twice a day. My doctor usually starts me on 2.5 mg drops twice a day when my levels go down. Testosterone pellets can be inserted in the buttocks for a slow, steady time release, lasting four to six months, if you don't want to take pills.

Testosterone cream is available from compounding pharmacies (see Resources, pages 347–348). It is applied in a small amount to the clitoris and the inner labia to help improve sensation. It also helps build up thin atrophic genital tissue. The cream is highly effective in increasing sensation during sexual stimulation. It's great for jump-starting things. You usually have to use it for a few days to a couple of weeks to get the feelings started. It's especially useful if your head has been full of all the things you need to get done, when the lists won't go away even though you try not to think about them. This cream puts you in the mood for love, and it really works. In addition, it's a wonderful lubricant, if that is an issue. As we get older and our hormones get out of balance, most of us experience some degree of dryness in the vaginal area. Testosterone cream helps greatly. Don't forget and think this testosterone is a magic cream, like whatever you put on your face at night to fight wrinkles. Your vaginal area will be moist again and your sex drive will return because you are balancing your hormones. The cream only jump-starts things. You need to be working on a larger plan to balance your hormones—testosterone is only part of the bigger picture discussed in the first part of the book.

Understand that it takes some time to achieve balanced hormones. After all, it took many years for your body to gradually lose its ability to make a full complement of hormones, so it will take a while to build these hormones back up to a full complement. During this time, testosterone cream is a godsend. Even after you have achieved hormonal balance, testosterone cream is something you may use occasionally when stress is a factor in your life. Nothing kills your sex drive like stress. Stress blocks hormonal production; so even if you are on hormone replacement therapy, stress can knock your levels out of whack until your doctor readjusts your dosage to compensate or until things in your life calm down. Your blood work will be a good indicator, but the way you feel is your best indicator after you have started replacement. You are not bugging your doctor if you call to ask about reactions to any new dosage. Your doctor can help you only if you work with him or her.

So keep a bottle of testosterone cream around, but understand that the need to use it is indicative of a larger issue. Something else is at work here. Use the cream to get you through this period, but don't come to depend upon it. One reason, of course, is that your hormones are out of balance—otherwise, you wouldn't need the cream—and the second reason is that using testosterone cream regularly will make you fat! Hormonal imbalance leads to weight gain. If you are using testosterone but your other hormones are not in balance, weight gain will follow. Notice the women who are regular users. Think about it—a lot of them are overweight. Why? For one thing, when your hormones are out of balance, you can become insulin resistant. This means that your cells, which comprise protein, fat, and carbohydrates, are loaded with all the sugar (from carbohydrates and foods that the body accepts as sugar) that your cells can hold. At that point, *any* sugars you ingest will be stored as fat. The most important element to remember is that testosterone, which is a hormone, needs to work in *balance* with the rest of your hormonal system. If you are giving yourself unnecessary daily doses of the cream because you think it will make you even hornier (which it won't), you will end up with increased levels of testosterone, which will put your other hormones out of balance. Hormonal *imbalance* creates weight gain because an imbalance of hormones makes you insulin resistant. So use the cream when necessary, but don't rely upon it or you will have trouble down the road.

It is your job to be attuned to your body's needs. Remember, no one will ever care as much as you do about getting it right. This is all about your quality of life. But when you have it right, everyone in your sphere will benefit. You are then able to be your "best self" in every way. You will exude happiness, security, and an overall sense of well-being. It is infectious. People will want to be around you so that some of what you've got will rub off. And you know what? It will.

ADRENAL BURNOUT

If you find that you are taking testosterone supplements and your sex drive is still not revived, then it is time to have your adrenals checked. There is a new saliva test that will accurately report not only your minor hormone levels, which include testosterone, but also your major hormone levels, which include adrenal, cortisol, and insulin levels.

Often when the body is under extreme stress, the adrenal and cortisol levels dip or, worst case, flat-line. As you have read in previous chapters, the adrenals are your major hormones along with cortisol and insulin. Without your major hormones you will not live very long. If your adrenals are low or flat-lined it will blunt not only your estradiol and progesterone levels but also your testosterone levels. No matter how much testosterone you are taking, it will not have an effect as long as your adrenals are blown out. This is a dangerous situation for your body. The symptoms of burnt-out adrenals are difficulty in sleeping, headaches, allergies, dizziness, and lack of a sex drive. If this resonates with you and you are taking testosterone supplements and still have low libido, most likely you have decimated your major hormones. Ask your doctor about taking the saliva test, because it will indicate whether you have blown out your adrenals.

Signs of menopause: You change your underwear after every sneeze.

10

DR. LAURA BERMAN: FEMALE SEX THERAPIST

I know they write songs about "doin' a-what comes naturally," but sometimes there are reasons other than instincts that interfere with a woman's abilities to have a healthy, enjoyable sex life. Dr. Laura Berman is a pioneer in helping women with sexual problems and their individual sexuality. I found talking with her not only revelatory but fascinating. She removes all discomfort and embarrassment from such a personal subject and allows us to explore those parts of our sex life that could be improved or maximized. Dr. Laura Berman has opened the Berman Center in Chicago to address the needs of those who desire counseling and help regarding the sexual part of their lives. She has also written a book with her sister, Dr. Jennifer Berman (see chapter 12), called For Women Only.

SS: Are women getting the optimum pleasure from their sexual relationship with either their spouse or their partner?

LB: We're working on it. In the beginning, so many women came to me and repeated over and over that they did not feel sexy or in the mood. In my practice I started to see patterns after talking to hundreds of women about their sex lives and about what went wrong. One of the things we started to see early on is that women—more often after their second child, but sometimes even after their third child—were experiencing low libido; and certainly there are a lot of social and psychological reasons why they would have low libido.

New mothers with a second child had to adjust to having a new member of the family. Taking care of the twenty-four-hour need machines that babies are, coupled with exhaustion, meant that they were not making sex their priority. Not that they didn't want it, but they were just too tired. But then, even after all of that had passed and they had plenty of child care and plenty of support, they still weren't feeling desire and felt flat sexually—they had no fantasies, no thoughts, no motivation. When we tested their testosterone levels, we found that they were extremely low. These were otherwise young, healthy women. We couldn't know if their testosterone was always low, but we did note that after the second child there was a change. I don't know if it is ovarian failure or some sort of evolutionary strategy—perhaps after having a couple of children we are supposed to focus on the offspring we have before we start making others—but we do know that a risk factor in giving birth can be resultant low testosterone.

SS: What is the most common complaint?

LB: The most common complaint is stress and depression. Women don't realize that our bodies are under chronic stress because we tend to put our own needs and our own emotional and physical feelings at the bottom of the totem pole. We have to get everything done first. So a lot of the time we don't even notice that we are having the physical symptoms of stress, or we can't do anything about the situation that is creating the stress. Women are working too hard, or balancing too much, or are in a horrible situation, but the majority of women will tell you that they experience stress on a daily basis and can't really get a reprieve from it.

SS: So does this chronic stress affect their hormone production? Is that why they have low testosterone?

LB: Yes, and the best explanation I have been given is that we used to think that everybody under stress experienced the "fight or flight" syndrome. What they found from a study at UCLA is that women do not go into fight or flight; we go into what we call the "tend and befriend" phenomenon—we want to turn inward, we want to nurture, we want to focus on our friends and family. We want to cuddle, but we don't want to have sex. Now if you think about it from an evolutionary perspective, they talk about the fight-or-flight response in terms of the caveman who is fighting off the saber-toothed tiger. With "tend and befriend," the women would go into the back of the cave and protect their children while the man fought off the tiger.

SS: What happens when you have chronic stress?

LB: There is a rise in oxytocin levels, which is our chemical of attachment. It is what we release from our breast-feeding. As our oxytocin levels go up, it creates a chain reaction that decreases the amount of free testosterone we have in our bodies.

SS: So that stress indirectly affects our testosterone production as well.

LB: Yes, but when you are thinking about younger women, the reason for a sexual dropoff is more often related to childbirth or chronic stress and depression than anything else. Of course, there are all the other emotional and relationship reasons, the most obvious being that your relationship is stressful, or your relationship isn't what you thought it would be, or your partner has gotten lazy, or you have gotten lazy, or you are too busy with the kids and work and everything else, and sleep is better than sex. All of those excuses are very real, but what I think creates a cascade of low desire is that women lose themselves, very often starting in their thirties, and become outwardly focused. One of the great things about aging is that when our kids leave home, we can really start to define and refind ourselves, and we can reach a sense of centeredness that we don't have when we are younger. Most young women start focusing so much attention on their family, managing their home, managing their kids' forty different after-school activities, cleaning the house, and all the things that they have to do that they lose sight of themselves in the process. In losing sight of ourselves—assuming there aren't other physiological factors—we tend to lose sight of our sensuality, our sexuality, and our energy, and we don't really take care of ourselves. We've been hung on by our kids all day long, we are stressed out, we see our partner at the end of the day, or we have been working all day and struggling to make ends meet, come home, and the last thing we feel like doing is having sex. It feels like another chore.

SS: That's interesting, because I interviewed a group of young working mothers, middle to late thirties, and they did refer to sex as "the dirty little chore."

LB: Yes, that is what they see it as, another chore they have to do. And their partners pick up on that. I try to counsel women and couples that they need to understand that it becomes a self-fulfilling negative cycle. As women lose interest in sex, for very real reasons—they are overworked and overtired, or there may be a hormonal or another physiological reason—they forget that for men the number one vehicle by which they achieve a sense of intimacy and connection to their partner is through being sexual. What happens when men are not getting sex is that they just inadvertently feel less close to their partner and less intimate. Therefore, they act in a less intimate and less connected way, even unconsciously. They are not doing it on purpose, but they don't think about doing the little things that mean so much to the woman.

SS: And then I suppose she becomes resentful or angry that he is not as close to her.

LB: Right; and when he complains about not having sex, she says, "All you care about is sex, and now you are not going to be romantic with me unless I have sex with you." Then she blames him for thinking only about sex when in reality the reason he is thinking about sex is not only because he wants to be sexual, and because he has the desire, but because he also wants to be close to her.

SS: Then what happens?

LB: He feels less close to her, he is less connected, he is less intimate; and because women are in large part inspired to be sexual because they feel close to their partners, she then shuts down even more sexually, and it becomes a vicious circle.

SS: I am exhausted listening to the cycle. As you were explaining I wanted to say, "*Stop!* Don't you see what's happening?"

LB: Sex feels like the dirty little chore for two reasons: one, because the woman is exhausted and it starts to feel like one more thing she has to do; and two, because she doesn't have the emotional and romantic context in her relationship to experience it as something pleasurable and loving and connecting. I don't think it starts out as a dirty little chore; I think it becomes a dirty little chore when the relationship begins to break down.

SS: Do you think that this is all part of the superwoman's desire to be perfect in everything she does? That she has lost sight of what is important?

LB: Yes. The quintessential modern woman has a career, a family, a beautiful home, and all of the material possessions she wants. In her spare time she gives back to the community and joins committee forums or alliances or whatever it is that she is interested in doing.

SS: So where in the world is she? Where is her center? Where is her identity?

LB: Everything she is doing is outwardly focused either on how she is perceived by others or on giving back to the community or to her family. Even exercise and nutrition for herself are more often about wanting to maintain a certain appearance than on enhancing herself, loving her body, or caring for her body. It is an outward focus, not an inward one.

SS: In speaking with women, I discovered that children are now sleeping in their parents' bed way too long; they are ages three, four, five, six, and older and still in their parents' bed.

LB: Yes, that is a big issue. Where there is a will there is a way to get the child out of that bed, unless it is a family who has a serious intellectual or emotional commitment to the family bed and believes that children should sleep with their parents as they grow up. But in families who are miserable, suffering with the child still in their bed, I look at that couple and wonder what purpose this child is serving. Usually one or both of them are relieved that the child is still in the bed and use the fact that the child is there as a way to avoid intimacy and sexual connection.

SS: But what about putting locks on the doors and having rules?

LB: They say they worry they are not going to hear their child, or they worry there will be an emergency, or they worry that an older kid might try to get into the room and see that it is locked and, God forbid, know what they're doing. They don't understand that the biggest gift they can give to their children is being open about the fact that Mommy and Daddy have an intimate relationship that is separate from the kids, and that they deserve privacy, and that their privacy needs to be respected.

SS: Where do you see this group down the road?

LB: Well, I think these women run a risk. It can go in two directions. More often than not, as a woman starts to reach forty and fifty she goes through a life crisis. Maybe her husband is cheating on her. Or maybe it is a child getting sick, or the child leaving for college, or a friend getting sick. Sometimes it is the woman herself getting sick. But something happens that will be a reality check to her—most often it is going through perimenopause. She will start to reorient herself and begin to turn inward a bit more and start to take care of her emotional self and her soul. But the problem is that these women run the risk of losing their partners, because as they start to go into this next passage, if the relationship has already started to disintegrate, they run the risk not only of the marriage falling apart, but also of the husband being more vulnerable to opportunities for infidelity, even if he is not seeking them out.

SS: So because he is starved for that emotional and sexual connection, he is much more vulnerable to other women.

LB: Yes, and these women want to give the connection to him.

SS: So let's go to the next group of women, who are my age, in their middle fifties, and in menopause. So many I have talked with are experiencing a lack of sexual feeling and no clitoral feeling, as though they are dead from the waist down. How much of this are you seeing?

LB: A lot of women come in complaining about this, and part of the problem is testosterone.

SS: Are you talking free testosterone?

LB: Free testosterone and testosterone in general. We have found that there are androgen receptors and genital sensation. When women have low testosterone, one of the signs, of course, is low libido, but it goes hand in hand with low genital sensation, low energy, and a low general sense of well-being. So we did sensory testing and found that women with low testosterone also had sensory impairment when we did sensory testing on their genitals.

SS: What causes the impairment?

LB: We don't know. We think it is because there are androgen receptors in the genital tissue, but we don't know what role they play. Is it for sensation, or does testosterone play a role in the nerve receptors so that nerve receptors without testosterone become atrophied? Because even when you replace testosterone, the sensation doesn't always improve as much as you would like; so is it because the nerve receptors have atrophied too long and they can't be resurged or revitalized?

SS: Can they?

LB: We only have our own anecdotal clinical experiences, but we have found that for women with low genital sensation and low testosterone, replacing their testosterone sometimes improves their sensation. Topical testosterone on the genital area or some other blood enhancers also seem to improve the sensation. The theory is that the increased blood flow pushes the nerve receptors closer to the surface of the skin, which makes them feel sensation better. So that is where Viagra and some of the other vasodilators have a role.

SS: Is there one perfect hormonal cocktail for every woman?

LB: No, every woman is different, so every woman has to find her perfect balance with the help of her doctor. It requires that the patient and the doctor work together as never before. What is likely is that as women go into menopause, with the help of their doctor they will devise the appropriate hormonal cocktail, which will hopefully include testosterone. Then, as needed, they can augment that with other medications, whether it be Viagra, one of the new incarnations of Viagra that are coming on the market, or some of the other arousal-enhancing agents that are out there.

SS: But Viagra does not put you in the mood, does it?

LB: No, but it improves genital sensation for women. You always have to be careful with hormones. Too much is not good, nor is too little. Testosterone gel or cream does get minimally absorbed into the system.

SS: But there are signs from using too much—facial hair, pimples, oily skin?

LB: Yes, so you will know if you're using too much. But testosterone creams and gels are also good for genital pain. We alternate with estrogen cream and testosterone cream because testosterone helps to toughen up the tissue as well as increase the sensation. There are other things to help also, like AndroGel.

SS: Can you give a list of what's available? Women are so reluctant to talk about this, but I know they are going to love reading about it.

LB: A good place to go is my Web site, www.BermanCenter.com. AndroGel is approved right now for men. It is a gel that is applied on a nonhairy part of their body. We use AndroGel as a last resort, if the woman is not responding well to oral testosterone or testosterone cream. But this medication is not dosed for women. It's not easy for us to use yet and is only available as an off-label prescription.

SS: Why are there no sexual medications for women?

LB: Until several years ago, women were not allowed to be included in any clinical trials.

SS: Why—are our genitals not as important?

LB: It's just the way it has been, but things are changing. Women are involved with the drug companies, so I believe in the next three to five years we are going to see a whole array of options that will enhance sexuality for women.

SS: Well, I hope so. Before I started to write this book, I always wondered why middle-aged men leave their middle-aged wives. It's not that they don't look great. I believe that as we go through the drastic changes of hormone loss, we behave badly because our chemicals are out of whack. We can't sleep, we're hot and then cold, we're tired all the time, we have strange itches, we break out in embarrassing sweats, we're bitchy, and we lose our sex drive. So after a while a man is going to say, "Who needs this?" and go out and find the new, improved, younger version of you.

LB: Right, but it's not so much of "Who needs this?" as something more subtle. Even with the nicest guys, their sense of self-esteem, their virility, their sense of masculinity, and their sense of attractiveness are all deeply tied to the women they love. So when they feel rejected, over time they just get more and more resentful. The majority of times when men have an affair, it has very little to do with the sex.

When a man is not having sex with his loved partner, it's because he is not feeling intimately connected with her, or appreciated, or loved, or attractive, or wanted, or desirable, or powerful, or any of those things he needs to feel good about himself. So if his self-esteem starts to dwindle, and then when he is at work or with his friends an attractive woman starts treating him as someone who is attractive and virile and powerful and whatever else, a part of him starts to wake back up.

SS: If the last resort for women is AndroGel, is it possible to bring a woman back to sexual life, or once you lose it is it gone forever?

LB: No, it is not gone. We have huge successes. The best success comes from a combined approach of medical treatment and talk therapy.

SS: Like what?

LB: Imagine a scenario where I'm talking to a perimenopausal or menopausal woman, and for medical reasons she has lost interest in sex, and the negative cycle we have been talking about exists. This condition affects the woman's self-esteem also. It affects the way she feels about herself, her body, her partner, and her relationship. Maybe there has been a rift that has been building in the relationship. So talk therapy helps the couple even if it is just getting over the awkwardness of trying to reconnect sexually. Between medication and talk therapy I would say that we have an 80 percent success rate helping women who come to us complaining of low or no desire.

SS: Tell me about your clinic.

LB: I am starting a new clinic in Chicago, offering not only medical treatment, but therapy as well, which means evaluating the couple's psychosexual history so that we get a sense of the relationship and anything that could be contributing to the problem now and in the past.

SS: Do you see them as a couple?

LB: We see the woman first individually. We spend around forty-five minutes with her, then we see them as a couple for another twenty-five minutes. They can come back for more couple sessions if necessary; but meeting them together helps us see what is going on with the couple, especially the man. This kind of therapy helps get both partners on the same page, and it helps alleviate some of the self-blame and mutual blame that they are putting on each other. This center is not only going to have ongoing individual and couples therapy as needed, but we will also have group couples, educational seminars, and physical therapy, so that when women have pain or atrophy in their genitals, we will be able to offer physical therapy to help them. We are also giving Pilates and yoga classes for strengthening pelvic floor strength. Pelvic floor strength is central to women's sexual function and starts to decline as we have children and then continues to decline. But pelvic strength is central not only to the woman's pleasure, but to her partner's as well.

Yoga and Pilates also give women an opportunity, as I was talking about earlier, to reconnect with their bodies.

SS: Well, I hate to be commercial, but that is a great use for the ThighMaster. One of its big benefits is its ability to strengthen the pelvic muscles.

LB: You know, you're right. I think I will start giving them out at the clinic.

SS: Let me ask you, aren't people embarrassed to go to a sex therapist?

LB: Well, it is a huge step for a couple to admit that they need therapy, but you would be surprised how many men call and want to make appointments for their wives. And men are so relieved that there is help available, and that we are not going to be telling them that it is all in their heads. We say to them, "Let's find out what is going on, let's look at the whole woman and see all the factors that could be contributing to her problem: the medical factors, hormonal as well as blood flow, and anything else that might be contributing from her surgical history, her past history, or any medications that she is on." We also look at her earlier sexual development, any trauma history she may have had, the messages she got about sex when she was growing up, how she feels about her body, how she feels about herself, how she is able to advocate for her sexual needs, whether she understands her body and how it works, what is happening in the relationship, what the level of communication and intimacy is, what the level of romance is, and what the level of affection is, because that is the thing that starts to go when the sex goes—they are not affectionate with each other anymore, and there are hurt feelings that need to be dealt with. You see, we can pump a woman full of all the hormones she needs, but if she is not feeling safe with her partner or connected to her partner, she is not going to be successful in her sex life.

SS: I have to say, I never knew that a sex therapist existed until I read your book.

LB: I've been working very hard to educate physicians, in particular gynecologists, because they seem to be the ones who hear a woman say as she is walking out the door, "Oh, by the way, I haven't wanted to have sex for over a year." So part of my work is collaborating with the doctors to effectively deal with women with their physical issues as well. The perfect balance is to have a sex therapist and a medical practicioner who specializes in this, and that's not easy to find.

SS: Where do we go if this is what we are looking for?

LB: There's my sister's clinic at UCLA, Dr. Jennifer Berman. There's the clinic I am opening in Chicago, and here and there, there are some doctors who have sex therapists working with them. Not many, but they do exist.

SS: As I keep telling my readers, this passage takes handling. It is really up to each woman to find the help she needs even if it means she has to drive long distances or fly somewhere. It's crucial to her well-being, her longevity, and her happiness. If a woman isn't willing to find the care she needs for herself, then she is going to end up taking an antidepressant to deal with her sexual dysfunction.

LB: Right, and then with the antidepressant her sexuality isn't helped, but she doesn't care. Then the antidepressant makes her sexual dysfunction worse. I don't understand it—there have been studies that verify antidepressants do not help with PMS and menopausal symptoms.

SS: Yes, and it seems like prescribing a Band-Aid to me.

LB: Yes, it is a Band-Aid. When someone is suicidal or unable to function, then there's a role for antidepressants. But the problem is that the primary prescribers of antidepressants are now primary care physicians. They're not doing any extensive evaluation or providing ongoing therapy to get to the core of why the woman's depressed. They're just putting a Band-Aid on it. When women have sexual problems where there may be very real emotional or physical causes, I say okay, but antidepressants are not always the answer.

SS: What needs to change relative to medical training?

LB: There is very little education about how to talk to patients about sex and about sexual medicine in general.

SS: Yet what makes the world go round?

LB: I know, it's very, very sad. Doctors don't get the education; plus our society is litigious, and because of this many doctors have told me that they are afraid to even ask a woman about her sexual function because she may think he is sexually harassing her, or she may think it's inappropriate.

SS: Are you able to work with other doctors regarding this?

LB: I have to find ways for them to indirectly open the doors so the patient can bring it up. But the other problem is managed care. A doctor has fifteen minutes to conduct the entire visit, so how can you open up that Pandora's box? Because even if it's a physical problem, and it's causing her tremendous distress, and it's the first and only time she has the courage to bring up that her husband is disconnected from her, and she's upset, and now she's crying—doctors don't want to open that up when they have twenty patients waiting.

SS: So what's the remedy?

LB: We have this course called "Women's Sexual Health, State of the Art Series." This year we had about three hundred people, mostly health care professionals, and our goal was to educate them about sexual medicine and how to get comfortable talking about sex, how to take a sex history, how to know whether a patient's a good candidate for medical intervention or better suited for therapy—things they should be taught in medical school. I also encourage doctors to visit our Web site, because it is intended not only for laypeople, but for doctors and professionals, too. This is working very well for us because it gives doctors a place to sort of pawn it off and not have to deal with it.

SS: How long can a woman remain sexual?

LB: Forever. There's no reason a woman should not be able to remain sexual; plus, sex will keep her healthy. Sex is one of the major things that keep us connected to ourselves. A woman who has a happy, healthy sex life feels happier in general, feels more feminine, more attractive and aware and connected to her body, which will allow her to be more aware when things go wrong with her body. You can be physically intimate and physically connected and even orgasmic until you die. I have a patient who is ninety-three years old. About five or six years ago I mentioned something about masturbation, and she said, "Oh, I never do that!" And I said, "Why not?" Her husband had died when she was in her sixties, and she hadn't been with another man since. "Oh, I wouldn't even know what to do," she said. So I said, "All right, I'm going to send you some stuff." I sent her a tiny purple vibrator (her favorite color is purple), and I included some diagrams showing her how to use it. A few weeks later she said to me, "You know that thing you sent me? It was a little small, don't you think?" So

I gave her a bigger one. A couple of months later, she mentioned that she had a second vacation home that she was going to and she asked if I could send one to her there also.

SS: So she's liking it, she's having fun. But for most people, buying a vibrator must be a very embarrassing thing. Where does one buy one?

LB: That's a good point. There are lots of options online. There's one site called www.grandopening.com and another one called www.goodvibes.com. Both of them are oriented toward women. Good Vibes, which is really Good Vibrations, is in San Francisco, and the cool thing is that they send orders in an unmarked package. It just says "Open Enterprises" or something. If you don't order from them for a couple of months, they drop you from their mailing list. The top site right now is www.drugstore.com.

SS: What role can a vibrator play?

LB: It plays more of a role than people imagine. As we start to age, sex gets harder for women, and they think of it as some sort of failure, as do men. My job is to ask or encourage them to include a vibrator in their sex life. It can be very beneficial. There's a whole range of vibrators that are very small. Some can actually fit between people and can be incorporated into sex, or a woman can have her clitoris stimulated to get things going, and those women who complain of feeling numb are able to jump-start their sexual feelings with clitoral stimulation from a vibrator. Even with testosterone cream or capsules or some of these other vasodilators or blood flow–enhancing agents, a vibrator can also help. Sometimes we need more sensation and more stimulation than when we were younger.

SS: So do you give a prescription for a vibrator?

LB: I do. When I am with a woman, we go over everything that's gone wrong and everything that's working and not working. Then I divide the treatment plan, which includes Kegels. But along with the other treatments, I will write down what vibrator I think would work for her, and what books and videos.

SS: Which videos and which books?

LB: There's a range. It depends upon what her issues are. If it's that her partner doesn't know how to stimulate her, and she doesn't quite know how to tell him, then we talk about books on sexual technique. If she feels sort of awkward because she was a virgin when she got married and doesn't really know how to pump things up, I may introduce her to books and videos on erotic massage or on spicing up her love life or things like that. If she's never tried self-stimulation, I might introduce her to a standard plug-in vibrator. If she can have an orgasm on her own but needs extra clitoral stimulation and can't have it during intercourse, then I recommend a smaller vibrator. There are different brands.

SS: Is there a G-spot?

LB: I certainly think so. There's a lot of controversy about what the G-spot actually is.

SS: It's on the inside wall directly behind the clitoris, isn't it?

LB: Yes, and many believe that the two are intricately connected. Many people don't realize it, but the clitoris goes up 10 cm inside. It branches out to where the pubic bone is located. So it actually has two arms that go way back inside the body. It's not only that external button you see. Often the G-spot is where the Skene's glands are in a woman, which is analogous to the prostate gland in the man.

SS: So are there vaginal orgasms as well?

LB: Definitely. Most women will report that vaginal orgasms are much more intense. They include pelvic floor and uterine contractions, and they feel much deeper than a clitoral orgasm. But what I tell people is that an orgasm is an orgasm is an orgasm. It doesn't matter. The majority of women do not reach G-spot orgasm. But I think Kegel strength has a lot to do with it.

SS: What part does a religious upbringing play in all of this?

LB: Religious interpretation is so often sex-negative, that sex is bad. A lot of women (and men) have been raised in an environment where their religious leaders told them they had to wait to be married before they had sex. This communicated that sex was wrong, or bad, or dirty. Masturbation was wrong, as was anything that could lead to a sexual energy or motivation because it might make you want to have sex before marriage. So these women have grown up with all these negative messages about touching themselves, about sexual pleasure, and about exploring sexuality, even with themselves. Then it's expected that on their wedding night they are just going to turn on a light switch and become a sexual being. Those messages, which basically have been the entire nature of their sexual development, are really difficult to turn off.

SS: What about childhood abuse? And I don't mean just sexual abuse.

LB: Anything that interferes with our development—our sense of being in control, our pride in our bodies, our pride in our accomplishments—or anything that interferes with the development of positive self-esteem and our ability to trust and make ourselves vulnerable can negatively impact our sexual lives. So if there is emotional abuse, physical abuse, sexual abuse of any sort, it will interfere with a child's sense of self, self-esteem, and body image and her sense of control and sexual development. Without that sense of self, she doesn't have the ability to enjoy sex and respond sexually.

SS: Do you think sex should be taught?

LB: Absolutely. I create sex education programs, not only for kids, but for parents, too, to teach them how to raise their children to be sexually healthy. In reality, sex education starts at birth, just with touch and sensuality. There are so many things you can do for your children: massaging your babies and helping them develop a sense of sensory awareness by encouraging them throughout their lives; praising them and encouraging them to have a sense of pride and joy in their bodies; allowing and not repressing their desire to explore themselves sexually; not slapping their hands and telling them that masturbation is bad. You may need to guide them to where it's okay to masturbate. You know, if you have company, then it's a good time to tell them, "I know it feels good, and it's fine to do, but it's really something you do in private."

SS: Where would you like to see people's attitudes about sexual therapists, about women and sexuality, go?

LB: I think women need a stronger sense of entitlement so that they feel they deserve a sexual response. It's worth seeking answers for. It has to be okay to seek help. In fact, seeking help has to become a good thing. Women have to realize they deserve to enjoy sex, and it doesn't mean you are a harlot or that something is wrong with you. It has to be okay to admit that sexual enjoyment is missing from your life and you want to do something about it. In the beginning when we first started this treatment, women would be cringing when they came in: "I can't believe I'm coming to a doctor's office about this." They were embarrassed that they were placing so much importance on their sexuality that they were actually seeing a specialist about it. But I'm starting to see a shift. Women are coming in now and saying, "You know what? There's help available and I'm going to take advantage of it." I would like to see more and more women feeling entitled to their sexual response and acknowledging that sexual response is a basic part of their general health and wellness. They have to stick to their guns when their doctors shuffle them around, or when somebody tells them that this is all in their head, or that this is not a big deal. I would like to see women hold on to themselves and find themselves. In order to do that, you need to keep yourself grounded against all the other pressures. Women have to be motivated and proactive right now, but in the future I'd like to see it come to a place where women don't have to be so intensely tenacious and motivated in order to get help.

SS: I guess at this moment it is necessary for women to be highly motivated. Motivation can save a marriage.

LB: Right.

SS: I believe the work you are doing will save marriages and families.

LB: I believe that it already has. It's very rewarding. If this center proves successful, we plan to open more in other major cities. But right now women have to be proactive—they have to do research, fight with their doctors, and keep asking the same questions again and again and again.

SS: This has been very enlightening. I always thought that sexual dysfunction was the domain of menopausal women. I had no idea how pervasive it is. But this generation is an amazing group of women. We were the women who came into our young adulthood in the sixties, the baby boomers. We are the first generation who wanted better communication than our parents had—we went to therapy, and we got to the bottom of the things that tried to keep us from being all that we could be. And now we've hit a new wall: a lack of understanding about menopause and its ramifications and effects. But the sky is still blue and hopeful because there are professionals like you to guide us and help us through.

LB: And I love what I do.

Perks of being over forty: In a hostage situation you are likely to be released first.

11

KAREN: A FORTY-YEAR-OLD EXPERIENCE

I wanted to talk with younger women, those still considering the possibility of having more children, those for whom menopause is a long, long way down the road, who are burned out because of the "superwoman" complex. They understandably want it all, but it appears there is a price. To be the perfect wife, the perfect mother, the supersuccessful businesswoman, to have the perfect house, give the perfect dinner parties, volunteer at school, bake cookies for the bake sale, give the perfect business presentations, and on top of all this be a sex pistol in the sack with her husband at the end of the day is exhausting, to say the least. There is not enough time in the day, month, or year to be all of the above. As a result, it seems thirty- and forty-year-old superwomen are exhausted. It is taking its toll physically and hormonally. Remember that hormone production is blunted by stress. The superwoman's life is so stressful that at the end of the day there is little to no energy left for sex. I suspect a good night's sleep is the most desirable item on the agenda.

Karen's story appears to be typical of what is going on in this age group with women who are superachievers. The surprising information is that the drive and the desire for sex are blunted by exhaustion and the resultant low testosterone and low estrogen that stem from the stress of this overactive lifestyle. Add to that the lists that occupy the superwoman's mind and it is understandable that something will have gotten off track. Of course, reprioritizing is essential, but in most cases that is not going to happen. What if hormone replacement could be the magic pill to get these women through this stressful and difficult time? This is Karen's story. I was exalted and exhausted after I finished speaking with her. She is bright and intelligent and has so much going for her, but the quality of her life is impaired by her body's physical inability to keep up, and it is working against her.

I am thirty-nine years old; by the time this book is published I will be forty. I had never given hormones much thought. Like most women, hormones were a mystery to be dealt with down the line— it was all about menopause, which didn't concern me and did not appear to be a particularly pleasant passage, so I thought it was better not to think about it until I had to.

The first time hormones became a living, breathing factor in my life was during pregnancy and nursing. It was the first time I realized that I was not in control of my body. It was as though I had lost part of my brain. I've always been so good at math; when out with my girlfriends, I was always the one who could instantly figure the bill, who owed what, factoring in that this one had to fly down so she shouldn't have to pay as much. This would take my brain an instant to decipher. But while pregnant, I couldn't remember a phone number. It was the first time I realized the powerful influence hormones had on my life.

When I was pregnant, I had an acute sense of smell. If my husband ate garlic, I had a difficult time sleeping with him. The smell nauseated me, made me really sick to my stomach. It was only in retrospect that I was able to put it all together, that it was hormonal and that the hormones were in control of my body.

Then there was the weight gain that hung around as a new layer, like another whole me, after the baby and throughout the entire four years that I nursed both my children. When I was going through it, I just presumed it was environmental, but as soon as I stopped nursing, everything came back into balance.

My personality changed during pregnancy also. I became very quiet. My husband would constantly ask if anything was wrong, but I just wasn't aware until looking back on it how inward I had become. It wasn't until afterward that I would think to myself, Ohhh, that's what it was. Once again, another awareness of hormones and that they were not just the concern of menopausal women.

There were the physical changes also. After four years of nursing, my breasts flattened out. In fact, my four-year-old started saying, "Mommy, your boobies look like socks." That was pretty depressing, but after about six months they puffed up again. Hmmm, another hormonal change; my hormonal balance was on a roller coaster. I was beginning to realize that hormones were in charge of me physically, mentally, and emotionally.

I experienced a severe drop in my sex drive. I had a hormone panel done by my doctor to find out that my lack of libido was due to a complete absence of testosterone. Frankly, I was relieved. I had been so distraught at my lack of desire, and now I knew it was physiological. My husband would come to me, but it was as though I were looking through a window. I wanted to have those feelings, but they just didn't seem attainable.

All of this is so difficult for me. I am a perfectionist—I want to be the best wife and create the best home for my family; I want to be the best cook and make crafts by hand; I want to be the best mother and prepare pure food for my children and make sure they feel loved and nurtured. When it comes to work, I am very task oriented. I can get it all done. Next! Bring it on! I love the challenge of watching the business we started grow into something so exciting and successful.

Around this same time, my husband and I spent two years remodeling our home while living out of boxes in a rental in which we had no interest. It was temporary, and we put our lives on hold while building our dream house.

The stress of remodeling, being the perfect mother, starting a new business, running to school with cupcakes for the class (home-made and decorated, of course), and giving the perfect dinner parties was taking its toll. Something didn't feel right. Never did I factor in that I was out of whack hormonally. I just assumed the anxiety was a normal part of everyday existence.

One day I went to the doctor (I have a great cutting-edge doctor), who did another hormone panel on me and thought there must have been some mistake because my adrenals were so high. "With numbers this high you must be a crazy person—you must be bouncing off the walls," he said. "I know it must feel great to be able to race through your day and accomplish so much, but it's going to catch up with you and you are headed for a big crash." It was a wake-up call, but one I didn't take all that seriously. I had a strange sense of pride that I could do it all. . . . But could I?

One evening my husband asked me for something, and I just blew up at him. It was irrational and emotional, and afterward I felt so bad because I love him so much. I felt terribly guilty that my need for perfection did not leave time for me to be the perfect wife for him. I mean, after my typical frenzied day, how am I supposed to jump in the sack and be the perfect lover? Something's got to give, and it was here that it was caving in.

My husband is very understanding. I don't have the same complaints I hear from my other girlfriends. My husband does pitch in. He shares responsibility for the children, he cleans up after dinner, and he is there for me whenever I need something. I began to think, How long will he wait for me to come around? My husband is the picture of health—he is an athlete, so he is in peak physical condition, and on top of that he is a hunk. How long can my excuses of being overworked and overtired and having too much on my mind remain viable? It makes me feel so sad. I don't know how to fix it. I know it's physiological, but for some reason I can't seem to accept the fact that I have to make some changes. I know I have to get my health on track, I know my hormones are out of whack, yet it's hard to make the connection that I might need hormone replacement in my life at this time. Somehow I feel as though I've failed if I have to supplement my hormones at this early age.

This scenario is no different from those of any of my girlfriends. They are all complaining that at the end of their busy, frenzied, hectic, overachieving days the last thing they feel like doing is having sex. One girlfriend refers to it as "the dirty little chore," like taking out the garbage. In fact, just yesterday she talked about how she "had to take out the garbage last night, ha ha ha." Twice a week she lets him have his way with her, to get it over with so that she can finally get some rest.

We're all working too much, we all have too much stress and anxiety, and we all have low libido. My sister said to me recently, "It's the ones who make their whole lives about their children who end up alone with their children." I don't want that, but I can see how easily it can happen. I feel so guilty. I know I am not meeting the needs of my mate.

I make feeble attempts to fix it. I went back to my doctor, and he gave me testosterone cream, but it made my skin rough and my face break out. I thought, Well, how sexy are pimples, so I stopped using it. My doctor said that obviously the dosage was wrong, but for some reason I didn't pursue getting the right dosage.

I know that I am not eating great. I grab food on the run during the day and take a bite here and a bite there. I know psychologically I am doing it because I can stay really thin this way. Being thin seems to be overly important, but when you are thin you look as though everything in your life is going right. I guess I want the outward appearance of my life to look perfect. Thinness does that.

Lately I have started to pad up a little bit. Not a lot, just five pounds, but it has me nervous. How can I be gaining weight when I haven't changed my eating? I'm sure at the bottom of it is some other hormonal change. Deep in my heart I feel that that little perimenopause is peeking its head out of the ground. I know I am not taking care of myself, and my excuse is that I don't have time. I have started exercising a little, and at the same time I am putting on a little weight. I can't figure out the connection between the two. I can just feel that my body is beginning to betray me.

I need to go to a spa. I need to go away with my husband so that we can just love each other and take care of each other. My husband is so great. He will do anything to get me in the mood. He'll give me a massage, he'll tell me I am so hot. He just loves me and my body. He thinks I am so juicy and great. But I find there just aren't enough hours in the day. It's so important for me to please everybody. I get depressed when I think I am slipping. I feel guilty when my husband and I go out for the evening, but I also feel guilty if we don't go out for a date. If the kids start acting out, then I feel that I am letting them down also.

Work can overtake my life. I could work 24/7 if I didn't have kids. I had my children later in life. I was in my mid-thirties, and the toll on me mentally and emotionally is exhausting. I look at other women who are in their late forties with children my age, and I think, How do they do it? It is a harder job the older you get. There is only so much energy. It puts the body through so much.

When my husband and I do make time for sex, it's so great. It creates a connection between us that lasts throughout the next day. It's the little looks we give each other—that knowing of the intimacy we shared. I want that with my husband, always. But life gets in the way; the stresses begin again, my mind gets full of noise, my anxiety increases, and then my hormone production goes wacky again. I am beginning to understand the connection.

I think it's classic with women my age. We have so much to prove, and we want to have it all. It's the superwoman complex, but it is taking its toll on our health and our relationships. I realize that my own self-maintenance is not high on my list. I know I need to get back to my doctor, but this time I am going to follow his program. He has been offering it to me, but I have been too busy to hear. It's a big commitment. I have to make some serious changes in my life to protect all that I value. I don't know why I am not at the top of my list. I don't know what drives me. It's such a cliché, but we all need to clone ourselves. The other day was so classic me. I had to go to a mother-daughter tea at two o'clock, and at one-thirty I was at a boutique hurriedly buying an outfit. I pulled it off, and I looked rather nice, but when I looked down at my feet in my new open-toed shoes, my toes were in bad need of a pedicure. I wanted to curl those things into my shoes, because now all I could see were my feet, which were in such need of some tender loving care. Instead of giving myself credit for getting to the tea at all with my schedule, I obsessed about my toes. That's my perfectionism driving me again.

I get depressed because it's all too much. I am aware that the stress is damaging me physically. I know I am not there for my beautiful husband. It's as though I am watching him go somewhere, and I'm not on that train with him. I have to get back on that pace with him. I don't want to end up this old haggard wife with the hot husband. My marriage and my relationship with my husband are so important. I have to start making us a priority. I am going back to my doctor. I'm gonna do it this time. I'm hearing myself talk, and it's clear to me that I am the problem. It's me, and it's my hormones. I need my doctor to help me get my life back on track. It's a lot of work, but if I don't do it and something happens to me, this whole thing I've worked so hard to create will crumble. What good is the perfect house, with the perfect children, and the fabulous business, without the stuff of life: contentment, relaxation, fun? I have forgotten about fun. I'm so busy being perfect that I have forgotten that life is to be enjoyed and to have fun.

I have to work on the addiction of work. I am addicted to adrenaline. I love being busy; I am stimulated when I have a hundred things going at once, but at what price?

If ever anything were to happen to my marriage, I would look back and remember when it started. The bitchy times, the short-tempered times, those "fly off the handle" moments. These are the destructive things that break down the best of things. I used to look at my sister and think, What's wrong with you? She was such a perfectionist. Now I've become her. I have to work at this.

I hope my story helps women in the same position. I never realized how serious this whole scenario had become until I started talking about it. We have to help one another. It will take a shift in my thinking, a reevaluation of my priorities, a realistic look at what I want and how can I have it all without sacrificing that which means the most to me. I want to get my life back on track. We women are mirrors for one another. Maybe by seeing my "chicken with her head cut off" existence, someone else will realize how crazy it all is. To think, it all might start coming together with a dose of testosterone.

KAREN: A FOLLOW-UP

I'm happy to report that before this book went to print I spoke with Karen again. She called to let me know that she really had made getting well a priority in her life. She went back to her doctor and had a full hormone panel run. Not only was she practically zeroed out on testosterone, but her estrogen was at half the level it should be for her age, and her progesterone was also low.

Her doctor prescribed natural bioidentical hormones in the form of creams. She's been on a low dose for the last three months and has this to report.

I can't tell you the difference this has made in my life. Within a couple of weeks I could see and feel the difference. Those extra few pounds I had started to carry began melting off. Finally, my body was responding when I was eating right and exercising. There is such frustration when you're doing what you're supposed to be doing and you're still not getting results. The hormones did the trick. But perhaps the greatest improvement is my mood! I am better able to handle the normal everyday stressors that come my way. My temper is much better and I don't sweat the small stuff. Before getting my hormones balanced, you could have told me all day, "Don't worry about it!" but my feelings were real and could not be discounted.

My husband and I started seeing a counselor just to protect what we have created. We made some headway, but once I started the hormones, we ran out of things to discuss! Our sex life has also improved. It's not yet back to full speed, but I've even initiated it a couple of times! My doctor told me that he has a therapist who sends patients his way from time to time. Once he balances their hormones, they usually stop the therapy! That's how powerful our hormones are to our everyday lives.

Thank you, Suzanne, from the bottom of my heart, for encouraging me to seek out these answers for myself. I have such a leg up on the next passage that will come my way. I plan to stay balanced and follow your lead. I love my cream! It's my happy cream, and I can't thank you enough for helping me to see that taking care of myself is the best way to take care of my husband, my children, and even my business. With much love, from a not-quite-cured perfectionist, but at least a much happier one!

Perks of being over forty:
Your investment in health insurance is
finally beginning to pay off.

———

12

DR. JENNIFER BERMAN: FEMALE SEXUAL DYSFUNCTION

Dr. Jennifer Berman is one of the few female urologists in the United States with specialized training in female urology and female sexual dysfunction. Sexual dysfunction is an embarrassing and uncomfortable condition, and there are very few places a woman can go to find answers. Dr. Berman provides a great service in a comfortable and safe environment. She has also written a book with her sister, Dr. Laura Berman (see chapter 10), called For Women Only.

At some point, most women will experience some sort of sexual dysfunction, usually because of hormonal imbalance, but until recently it has never been given any importance because women are still able to function even if they don't feel anything. I asked her, "What percentage of women in this country are unfulfilled sexually, and why?"

JB: I guess that would really depend upon what range you are talking about, but overall anywhere between 30 to 50 percent of American women have complained of sexual dysfunction at some time in their lives.

SS: What are the reasons?

JB: The reasons are multifaceted and can range from emotional, relational, and psychological issues all the way to hormonal, medical, and surgical.

SS: What are the most common complaints?

JB: The most common complaint that women relate to their sexual dysfunction is low desire. Again, the reasons for that can be medical and/or physical, but often it is a combination of the two. Even if the original problem is physical, emotional and relational problems can result. And vice versa. If a women comes in because her relationship is in crisis and she is not satisfied with her marriage, frequently we will find that there is also a hormonal problem or some medication that she is on or has been on in her medical history.

SS: What is the average age of your patients?

JB: The average age of the women I see in my practice is forty-five, so they are perimenopausal; but I also see older women and menopausal women. Problems begin around the age of forty-five, but some women will start to notice changes about themselves in their late thirties and early forties. My mission is to inform and educate women about the potential changes that can happen so they can be in tune with their bodies.

SS: How does a woman know when she is in menopause? A lot of the same symptoms are present when a woman experiences PMS or perhaps is just having a bad day.

JB: Very often, women will start to experience changes in their hormones, whether it's irritability, or not sleeping as well, or that their memory is not quite what it used to be. They may experience vaginal dryness, low libido, lack of sexual response, and a lack of feeling in the genital area.

Most often, the problems are due to subtle, if not dramatic, changes in hormones, but I cannot say 100 percent that is the reason all women experience problems. There can be other emotional relationship factors; and a woman will say, "I feel tired, I feel like I have low desire, I feel like I don't respond very well." Yet when she is on vacation in the Caribbean without the kids, just she and her husband, everything is fine. For her problem to be defined as hormonal, it has to cross through all situations and be persistent and pervasive.

SS: Is stress a major factor?

JB: Stress is a major factor affecting women and their sexual lives and, for that matter, their emotional and physical lives also. Stress affects hormones. Stress in women can lower testosterone levels and cause libido problems and sleep problems. But sexual problems can also be caused by surgeries that result in nerve damage, such as in a tubal ligation. There is very little data in the medical literature to support this theory, but women would tell me that after they had their tubal ligation, they noticed their libido and their orgasms changed. I am not saying there is any science to support this, but we are definitely hearing this repeatedly from women.

SS: Are women experiencing lack of libido only in the case of tubal ligations, or would other surgeries cause the same thing?

JB: Any pelvic surgeries that impact blood flow and nerve supply to the genital area can affect a woman's sexual drive, including hysterectomy, removal of the uterus and/or ovaries, bladder surgery, or colon surgery.

SS: That is frightening. I've never given a thought to the fact that any type of pelvic or uterine surgery would have an impact on my sex drive.

JB: Many doctors still do not understand the dangers inherent to nerve and blood flow to the genital area during an episiotomy, which is a "taken for granted" procedure in childbirth. There are now different philosophies on the benefit of this procedure. Is it better to have a natural tear, or is it better to have a surgical straight tear? An episiotomy incision can definitely cause pain problems that will affect women throughout their lives. They come in and need revisions of their episiotomy scars or other surgical repairs, so it is important for women to know that these procedures can cause pain and nerve damage down the road.

SS: Did you start out wanting to specialize in women's sexual dysfunction?

JB: Yes, but when I first started my practice I thought sexual problems would primarily be the domain of aging and menopausal women. Now that I am immersed in this field, I am finding that younger women are experiencing sexual problems as well, and it is most often due to hormones. Even very young women in their twenties who are on birth control pills will and can experience libido problems and vaginal dryness, and they have no idea what is wrong with them. They go to their doctors and are told it's all in their heads. The birth control pills alter their hormones, and this is where the difficulty occurs.

Often in their mid- to late thirties, women experience testosterone deficiency syndrome, especially after having babies. It happens sometimes after the first baby, but more often after the second baby. Women will come in and say, "Life is great—I've got health, the kids are in school—but I still have this loss of desire and a dramatic change in feeling sexual. It just does not make sense that it is all because I am stressed and tired." In testing, I have found that they do in fact have low testosterone levels and do respond to testosterone. Some young women also have changes in their estrogen levels, so we now realize that after a first or second child, a woman's testosterone levels can drop so much that they need testosterone replacement forever. There is also a drop in progesterone levels, but that is temporary. There are dramatic fluctuations in a woman's hormones after delivery. But then, in theory, you are supposed to come back to normal and reequilibrate. Now, granted, normally estrogen and progesterone come back, and women do begin to menstruate again and start having normal regular periods and get pregnant again, but testosterone does not return in all women.

SS: How does a woman find out?

JB: I test through blood work. This is definitely not "one dose fits all." Some women do better with topical creams, some with oral sublingual delivery, and some with a gel. Each woman absorbs differently and responds differently. Right now, unfortunately, there is not an FDA-approved treatment plan or delivery system for testosterone in women.

Research is still ongoing, but doctors are now prescribing testosterone off-label and compounding. But one thing to bear in mind is that each compounding pharmacy is different. Doctors need to analyze which ones are better and which compounds work better.

SS: Most women would not think to go to a urologist for sexual problems. The natural choice would be their gynecologists.

JB: The doctors who have the greatest grasp on hormones are endocrinologists or reproductive endocrinologists. As a urologist, I had to learn about it myself. I went to meetings, I read, I talked to everybody, listened to everyone's opinion. I read the medical literature, I read the package inserts, I tried different ones and came up with what I felt comfortable doing. But there is no consensus on what every woman needs, nor, for that matter, should there be, because every woman is different and every woman metabolizes hormones differently and everyone responds to hormones differently.

SS: So you're saying that women have to seek out the right doctor for themselves, and that doctor has to be a self-starter and interested in the newest thinking relative to sexuality and hormones?

JB: Absolutely. When it comes to the correct doctor, women have to be on the prowl, because unfortunately, sexual dysfunction and hormones are not given much attention in medical school. Hormones are very complex. There is a lot to understanding them. You treat full-blown menopause one way, but women in perimenopause—say, in their forties, who are still getting a period and still have some estrogen levels—have to be treated differently, and this brings up a whole other issue. When do we start? Do you start when you are already there and having hot flashes, or is it better to start it earlier?

SS: No wonder women are so confused.

JB: Right, but women have to take charge of their bodies. Maybe they are trying but are not getting answers from their doctors. Women need to feel entitled and valued, to feel that their sexual health is important and that sexual dysfunction is not normal.

SS: So what do we do? Is there Viagra for women?

JB: There is no female Viagra at the moment. They are developing it, but in reality it will be the same for women as it is for men, just packaged differently. Viagra doesn't put you in the mood; but if you are in the mood, it works great. In women it induces warmth, tingling, and a pleasant feeling in the genital area. Women have reported that it does make it easier for them to have an orgasm and improves the intensity of orgasm, but it is not a libido pill. When I prescribe Viagra for a woman, I tell her that it requires stimulation either with themselves or with their partner. It takes thirty to forty-five minutes to work, and during that time, it's important to force stimulation through foreplay, kissing, or whatever it is that they do.

SS: Is Viagra the only way for a woman to jump-start her sexuality while she is working at getting her hormones balanced?

JB: There is also a device called Eros-CTD developed by a company with the intention of improving genital blood flow. It is basically a sucking vibrator, so it's an erotic aid as well as a physical stimulator, the premise being that if you can improve genital blood flow, you can improve sexual pleasure. The same principle applies to women as to men: Use it or lose it. The more sexually active men are, the more blood flows to the penis, and the fewer vascular changes and fibrosis that occur. It's the same for women. It begs the question, do you need an Eros or can you just have a healthy sexual life and/or vibrator to achieve the same effect? The Eros works best if you use it every day. I don't sell the machine in my office, but the erotica shops have done the $30 knockoff. Eros is made by a company called UroMetrics. But most women are uncomfortable with the idea of buying a device, so I have found that giving permission and a prescription to buy a vibrator has been very liberating. But if this does not help, medications and exams are crucial to be sure that damage has not been done to the blood flow to the area.

SS: Does intensity of feeling change as you age?

JB: As you get older, orgasms diminish in intensity, but this is hormone related. It is crucial to get blood levels to rectify this matter. Some women are able to have multiple orgasms, and others cannot. I don't have an anatomic or medical explanation of why this is so. But in theory all women have the capacity to learn to have multiple orgasms and also to ejaculate.

SS: Is it simply "doing what comes naturally"?

JB: Unfortunately, there is no school to teach sexual technique. It is very important for women to know what pleases them and how to stimulate themselves and what they like and what they don't like in order to communicate that to a partner. Men intrinsically don't know what to do. They learn from the women they have been with, but it is up to us to know what feels good and what doesn't and to communicate that.

Doctors can do only so much, so often doctors ignore women's sexual complaints for a variety of reasons. Perhaps it is because their education in medical school was lacking in that regard, or they are uncomfortable talking about these issues, or perhaps they don't have a treatment for it. Doctors like to be able to fix and treat problems. Unless they have a treatment or a solution in hand, they don't want to go there.

I do feel that doctors who use antidepressants as a remedy are doing so basically to shut the woman up. But then the woman's sexual dysfunction gets worse and she gains weight and then (usually) thyroid problems arise.

SS: What else is out there to help with sexual dysfunction?

JB: There is an herbal remedy called yohimbine, which has been out for a long time for men with erection problems, and it's just recently been looked at as a potential remedy for women. A lot of women have had some success with that. There is also a product called Xcite that has three herbs in it. I was approached to help design a placebo control study, and the study found that it was really effective. Since then I have prescribed it to a lot of different women, including my mother, who has breast cancer and doesn't want to take hormones. She said that for the first time in twenty-five years, she's having regular sexual dreams, she's having orgasms in her dreams, she's lubricated, and everything else.

SS: So what's in the future? Is there light at the end of the tunnel?

JB: Hopefully, the future will bring heightened awareness relative to sexual dysfunction. Women need to become aware of these problems and demand they get the care they deserve. This generation of women is different from my mother's and her mother's. They don't just sit back and take it and say, "This is what happens when you get old, so you'd better get used to it." I think there will be some sort of grassroots movement of women forcing the health care field and health care professionals to address these problems, to research these issues, and to develop appropriate therapies, both hormonal and nonhormonal. Women need to be proactive about their health, especially their sexual health, because it's not likely that their doctor is going to say, "By the way, how are you doing in that respect?"

SS: This has been very enlightening. Thank you so much.

JB: Thank you for doing this. A book like yours is going to help women through their confusion.

Perks of being over forty:
You quit trying to hold in your stomach, no
matter who walks in.

———

13

PATRICIA: A FIFTY-YEAR-OLD EXPERIENCE

Patricia is experiencing menopause and is not taking hormones. She did not want to take synthetic hormones because she has read of the problems that accompany taking these drugs. She would like to take natural hormones, but she is not able to afford them. Because your average gynecologist is not well versed in hormones, there is a lot of guessing going on in doctors' offices. When a menopausal woman comes in visit after visit, complaining about the symptoms, the doctor doesn't know what to do. Patricia's doctor prescribed what has now become a commonplace and accepted remedy. Instead of replacing the lost hormones with natural bioidentical hormones as determined by blood work, her doctor put her on an antidepressant. This is a Band-Aid that temporarily makes the woman feel better because her mood is elevated and the symptoms are more tolerable; but because the hormones are not being replaced, she is experiencing hormonal imbalance, which is accompanied by considerable weight gain. Patricia is a small person by nature, and the weight that is part of this passage is very depressing for her. In addition, the antidepressant she is taking brings with it a lack of zest and lethargy that is part and parcel of the strong drug. The combination of her lack of hormones and the effects of this drug is not making for an enjoyable passage. Her story is one of the more common for the average woman.

I am fifty-one years old as of next week. I am in menopause, but I am not taking hormones. I take isoflavones and phytoestrogens every day. They help a lot with the hot flashes. I also use progesterone cream to help me get through this difficult time. It's a cruel time of life. I mean, you are dealing with the empty nest syndrome, and then all these changes start happening to your body. When I entered menopause, I felt the whole thing was very unfair, but now I am getting used to it. I first realized something was changing when my periods became irregular. Coupled with that, I started experiencing a lot of anxiety—I had a racing heart and palpitations. I was really frightened that I was having a heart attack. It was an irrational fear, but I was feeling irrational pretty much all the time. The hot flashes were awful. I couldn't sleep because of them, and I felt depressed and very tired. Then I started gaining weight, and that was very distressing. Weight can really make you feel awful. On top of all this, I lost all interest in sex. The vaginal dryness made sex painful even if I had wanted it. I didn't want to complain because I had been avoiding sex for so long, but there was nothing I could do but yell, "Ouch!" I missed the closeness together. I worked all day, and I wanted to be with my husband in the evening, but with my moodiness, depression, vaginal dryness, and lack of interest in sex, I was not the most pleasant person to be around.

To make matters worse, my husband is also going through something neither of us understands. He's depressed about the empty nest, he doesn't like his job anymore, and he's tired all the time. His doctor recently put him on an antipsychotic drug. Between the two of us, it's pretty sad. What's difficult is that we really love each other. We are committed to sharing our lives together, but I want a better quality of life. When he's on the antipsychotic, he might as well not be home. He's just not "there." Maybe it has to do with low testosterone, I don't know—our HMOs do not pay for psychological or any kind of hormonal panel to be done, so we just guess at it and anesthetize the depression with prescription drugs.

I keep asking myself, Why does it have to be this way at this time in our lives? We've raised our kids—why do we have to put up with this crap now? This is a very hard time to get through together.

I am interested in natural hormones (real hormones), and I visited a pharmacist at a compounding pharmacy in my area, and he was wonderful. He sat with me for a full hour and explained about real hormones. My HMO will not pay for an endocrinologist, so I went to my gynecologist, and he put me on an antidepressant, Paxil, so I could handle the symptoms better. Believe me, I feel a lot better on the antidepressant, but I also feel angry that I am denied access to real hormones because I can't afford them.

I am still gaining weight. My body is so foreign to me at this time. I miss being thin. I still feel healthy and strong, but now my thyroid is acting up, so my doctor put me on thyroid medicine. At first I tried kelp because I had read about it, but I had a bad reaction, so I resigned myself to taking the thyroid drug. Add to this the absent-mindedness and the joint pain, and some days I want to scream. I take Premarin vaginal cream, and that seems to help with the other uncomfortable symptoms, so I'm doing the best that I can.

I've been in menopause for a year and a half. Things are better now than they were—they would have to be, given how horrible menopause was when it first started—I can't say this is the best time for me. I want all of this to be over. I want my old life back: the zest, the fun.

There are some good things about this time also. I feel the empowerment of this age. I went out and bought myself a new car. It may not seem like a big thing, but it was for me. I bought it with my own money, and I handled the entire transaction by myself. My husband usually does things like that, but I needed to do this on my own. I am no longer tied to my children. I see them, we are close, but I don't need to chart out each and every moment of their day any longer. I know there is an energy about this age, and if we women could harness it, I know it would be very potent. It's just that the hormones make it very confusing. At times my mind goes completely blank.

I've taken the attitude that I will get through this. One of the things about us baby boomers is that we are helped by one another. We will be very useful to our daughters and granddaughters. I want to be open with my daughters, and I want to tell them that everything is going to be okay. I want to share my knowledge, but this passage is a tough one. I hope they will have it figured out by the time they are going through this. It upsets lives, it upsets the balance, and it forces a change upon you that I wish would go away, but it won't, so we just have to get through it.

Perks of being over forty:
Your eyes won't get much worse.

—

14

ATHENA: A SIXTY-YEAR-OLD EXPERIENCE

Athena is a dear friend of mine. She has chosen not to take hormones of any kind, but because she is conscious of and proactive about her health, she is having an easier time of it than some of the other women who have gone the same route. She is happy and upbeat all the time. Hormones are a personal choice, and here is how she is coping with this passage. I ask you to decide for yourself if her way is the direction you would choose. She is enjoying a quality life, but she is experiencing symptoms. We talked on the phone, and here is her take on life at this age.

Actually, I'm fifty-nine, but who's counting? Fifty-nine, sixty—it's all great. Besides, what choice do you have? I love sex. I have always loved sex; and even at my busiest, sex was never my problem. It was always my destressor. So I guess I have been blessed with a healthy libido. I never thought it was unusual; it was just the way it was. I never had a problem with orgasms; in fact, I am the queen of multiple orgasms. My body has always been a willing participant. I used to hear women saying that lubrication was a problem. Well, it had never been a problem for me, but now it's a problem. In fact, I keep yelling when I am with my boyfriend of seventeen years, "My pussy is broken!" You get older, things change. . . . not my sexual desire, just my body's willingness to take part the way it used to.

I have chosen not to take hormones for two key reasons. One, I am generally a naturalist. My instinct is to let nature take its course. I realize at this age things are changing, but because I have enjoyed a great sex life thus far, I don't want to interfere. I understand that we are living longer and all that, but it doesn't feel right to me to try to alter things.

A few years ago, when I was fifty, I did try natural hormones: DHEA, estrogen, and progesterone. I hadn't yet stopped my period, but I was going to a "new thinking" kind of doctor who was of the mind-set that taking hormones was preventative, and I wouldn't have to entertain any of the nasty effects of menopause. I was on these natural hormones for a year and a half (my doctor never ordered a blood test), but it activated a regrowth of my fibroid tumors, which is why I had originally contacted this doctor in the first place. So now I have a mistrust of tampering with nature.

Second, I realize my decision is a trade-off. I know the great good feelings that come with balanced hormones, in particular the well-being that comes with natural hormones, but I don't want to have a period. It's just not a price I am willing to pay.

I am now in menopause. It came late for me, when I was fifty-eight, and my body is experiencing it, that's for sure. But the most upsetting aspect for me is lubrication. The well has run dry. I once was like Bahrain, an oil-rich country, but now I have to use vaginal lubricants, and I'm not crazy about this part.

I experience night sweats on a semiregular basis, but it doesn't drive me up a wall. I haven't lost my breasts as some women do, because I never had any. When God was passing out breasts, I was in the cafeteria eating lasagna. I do exercise. I have been going to an exercise class three times a week for ten years now. So my muscle tone is good, my weight is good, and my energy is good. I take very good care of myself, and I think this is the payoff. I'm in a good mood most of the time; in fact, I would say my mood is wonderful.

I started my period early in life, when I was twelve years old, and I went into menopause late. I think this has been an advantage. In total I have had more than my share of estrogen—according to my doctors, more than most women—but on the negative side I think this also explains my fibroid situation, which has plagued me. Because of this wealth of estrogen, I don't really relate to most women's complaints. I have had good fortune, but I have also been extremely proactive about my health all my life. I believe fully in the mind-body connection, so I also take very good care of my thoughts. I have always kept a good attitude, I do spiritual work by reading books that inspire me to be a better person, and I have wonderful friends. I am loving my life.

Do I feel fifty-nine? Yeah, I have muscle aches I never had before, and there is that vaginal lubrication situation, but I still love sex with my boyfriend. It's just a little more difficult at point of entry. My gynecologist has prescribed some kind of Pennzoil for the pussy, some kind of vaginal cream, and it's actually pretty good. Let me put it this way: I travel with it. I pack my toothbrush, my pajamas, and my v-cream.

As far as other symptoms, I think I may be a little more jittery and nervous. I have to watch that jumpiness because I just found out I have high blood pressure. I don't like that.

I have always slept well, like a baby, and now I find I get up at least once in the night to pee, but I go right back to sleep. It's a blessing to sleep soundly; in fact, it's a marvelous experience. I'm feeling really good, especially since my doctor had forecast that I was going to have an awful menopause because I was so estrogen rich. I'm glad to say he was wrong, although this is only my first year.

I think it's genetic. My mother did not have a traumatic menopause. She's eighty-nine and still full of energy. According to her, it occurred with no fanfare. It just wasn't a big deal.

When you reach this age, it's hard to know if it's just natural aging or hormonal deficiencies. Now, if I had lost my sexual feelings, as so many women report, I would probably rethink it with someone like Dr. Schwarzbein. You see, I spent years having heavy (and I mean heavy) periods. I had an arsenal of Kotex pads. Tampax couldn't hold the river that flowed from me each month. My periods had been a whole piece of my life, and it was burdensome. So that's why it's difficult for me to entertain the idea of starting up again with the whole period thing.

My skin is drier now, I am using a lot more moisturizing cream on all parts of my body, especially my arms and legs, but I'm not irritable, so it's an okay trade-off.

I am very sensitive to anything artificial. I am careful as to what I put in my body. I don't take over-the-counter drugs if I don't have to, and prescribed drugs are often difficult on my system. When I was on hormones, I got fatter and bloated, and I hated the feeling. I have been blessed with a healthy body, and I value that. I listen to my body and am vigilant about listening to the inner talk. I have friends who take sleeping pills and Prozac, and I wouldn't be interested in anything like that.

My big problem is constipation, but it's been that way since I was thirty years old. I know it's strictly from stress, but I have recently found an interesting acupuncturist/herbalist who is a naturalist, so now we are working on my "inner landscape" through herbs. I am taking enzymes along with the herbs, which help to absorb all the nutrients.

I am distressed about my high blood pressure. I think it's from my stock market losses, even though I am told it's genetic; but nonetheless I am on drugs, and I am not happy about that. I take beta-blockers, atenolol and Norvasc, for blood pressure, and a diuretic, hydrochlorothiazide. My bone density is still good; I mean, there is some loss, but not an alarming amount. I take a potassium enzyme for my bones, along with magnesium, potassium complex, vitamin C, something called Digest, and protease, which cleans the body of plaque.

I am paying attention to the high blood pressure because my dad had it, and so does my sister. It's impossible to discern how our earlier years affected us. I grew up in a very upset household. My father was a frustrated, angry man. He was yelling all the time; so today, when things go wrong, I have this feeling that the sky is falling. I have relearned; I have tried to accept the flaws and then fix them. I am into biofeedback as a result. I realize I can change my inner terrain, as well as help my body retrain itself to be calm. I am learning not to sweat the small stuff. My boyfriend has quiet confidence. He is a calm person, and he has been so good for me in so many ways. Over the years we have grown in intimacy. We are great companions, and we are very loving.

I believe women need to participate in their wellness at all levels. This passage takes managing, and those who do manage it have a better quality of life. If your life is not working, do something about it. I have an ex-mother-in-law who has hated her marriage all her life. She just can't stand being in the same house with her husband. And guess what? Her back is riddled with pain. But she is driven by "what would people say?" Also, she's of a generation of women who didn't drive, so there is no independence. I think that is why so many women my age are managing their pain with Prozac—they'll take anything to deaden the pain.

I'd like to say to women my age that we are in charge of our lives. I believe we have the power within us to alter our thinking, our outlook, and our habits. I also know that what we eat or drink has everything to do with our bodies and our wellness. We are far more in charge of our lives than we suspect. No matter how out of control or hopeless your life may seem, it is not out of reach for anyone to become increasingly happy and healthy.

At fifty-nine, I'm not only flying high, but I'm getting ready to fly higher. I have made a list of goals for the coming year. My business coach told me to write it down. My goal for this year is to become a sensational sixty! You cannot wait for other people to give you your kudos. You've got to say it yourself, kind of a verbal high five. Stop saying those things you constantly say to yourself on a daily basis—you know, the I can'ts. Start acknowledging the good things of each day, even if it's "I made a great poached egg this morning," and then say, "Atta girl."

PART III

LIFE
on your
own terms

Perks of being over forty: You can sing along with the elevator music.

15

QUALITY OF LIFE

Now that you are beginning to understand the importance of balancing your hormones for your physical health, let's look at the emotional and psychological benefits, too. When you are balanced, you are better equipped to take an honest look at your life and determine if you are living your life on your terms. This is the last chance to make changes. These can be tough issues to tackle. When your hormones are out of whack, taking on emotional issues can be devastating. We all know that the PMS-y time of the month is no time to deal with those things that have been on your mind and bothering you. Being chemically altered by PMS clouds your thinking and judgment. There is a tendency to overreact emotionally. Factor in hormone imbalance and life problems as we get older, and forget it. You will get emotional and never be able to make your point because your reaction will be so over the top.

·But you are entering the second half of your life, and I mean the second half. Do you want fifty more years of the same? Are you happy with the choices you've made for yourself? Are you in good health? If not, what are you going to do about it? You have a whole life ahead of you. You're not "too old." If life hasn't brought you all that you've wanted, this is your opportunity to make changes. This is your chance to reinvent yourself. I've had to do this several times in my personal and professional life.

I remember the most blatant "opportunity" came after being fired from *Three's Company,* a television show I starred in during

the 1970s. My five-year contract was up, and I went in to renego-
tiate (which is customary in the industry) and asked to be paid
what they were paying the popular men on television. For instance,
Alan Alda, who was starring on *M*A*S*H,* which was number
ten in the ratings, was earning eight times more than I was. My
show was number one, so I figured that my demands were not
unreasonable. Little did I know that the network had decided to
make an example of the next actress who asked for a pay raise, so
that other women wouldn't get the same idea that they could be
paid the same as men. Suddenly I went from starring on the number one show in the country to being unemployed and persona non
grata in the television industry. I was labeled "trouble," so no one
wanted to work with me. I became depressed and wasted my days
flogging myself for having been stupid enough to ask for such a
pay increase. I moped and felt sorry for myself for the better part
of the year until one day a little voice inside my head said, *Why are
you focusing on what you don't have? Why don't you focus on
what it is you have?*

Suddenly I had an awakening. What I had was enormous visi-
bility; everyone in the country knew my name. That was valuable.
What could I do with that? That's when I decided to become mul-
tidimensional. I took my well-known name and put together a
nightclub act. I worked night and day learning to dance, sing, and
work on material. I tried out the act for the first time in Denver,
and it was pretty dismal. The reviews were devastating. One
reviewer said, "Then she sang 'I Don't Know Why,' and I still don't
know why." But I had bookings at other places, so I was unable to
give up. It didn't take long, though, before the reviews were filled
with "charming" and "refreshing" and "engaging." I had reinvented myself as a nightclub performer. I stayed on the road for
most of the 1980s.

That's when I started writing books. I had nothing to do during
my days because I worked at night, so I decided it was finally time
to explore the effects of living my entire childhood with my violent, abusive, alcoholic father. As I wrote I was amazed at what I

remembered: the sounds, the smells, the weather, what we ate, what we wore. I remembered my mother's anguished cries; I remembered the fear I felt at the anticipation of the coming night's events. Who would be "it" tonight? Who was going to be the object of his rage? I remembered hoping it wouldn't be me, then the guilt I felt when it was my mother or my brother or my sister. I worked on the book every day for a year. One day I came to the end of the story. I had done it. I was now a writer. I had reinvented myself again. Now I had two careers.

The book, *Keeping Secrets,* came out and was a nationwide bestseller. My secrets divulged were no longer a source of pain and shame for me; rather, they became a connecting force with the people of this nation. I wasn't alone with my secrets, as I had always thought. I now knew that others had lived similar lives because my book prompted them to write to me and share their own secrets. Most of the letters started with "You've written my life story." So many letters came into our office that we could have filled a small room from floor to ceiling. As a result, offers for lectures came pouring in.

"I can't speak before people," I told my husband.

He booked me anyway. "I know you, you'll figure it out," he said.

My first lecture was dismal. I came equipped with fifty or so notecards, and people were literally falling asleep. I had been afraid to speak extemporaneously, so I relied heavily upon my notes, lost my place several times, and in general was pretty awful.

"I never want to do this again," I said to my husband, feeling humiliated.

"Well, we've already got three bookings that are not cancelable; so you'll have to do these, and then I won't take any more bookings," he said.

I was overwhelmed with fear. I didn't want to bomb again. Then the little voice inside my head spoke to me once more: *The notes didn't serve you well. Why don't you just tell the truth and speak from your heart?* After all, I had lived this story—why couldn't I just tell it as it happened? I had nothing to lose. It couldn't be any worse than this last experience.

Wow! What a difference. The audience was rapt. They listened to every word, and I received a standing ovation. That's when I realized that the truth is mesmerizing. You can't fail when you are telling the truth. There's no way you can get tripped up. Now I had a third career. The offers for lectures came pouring in.

In 1986 I was named Female Entertainer of the Year in Las Vegas along with Frank Sinatra, the Male Entertainer of the Year. I felt pretty good about that. I had reinvented myself. One night my husband and I were coming home from one of my shows in Las Vegas, and I found myself imagining our lives down the road, twenty or thirty years or so. It was clear that singing, dancing, and entertaining night after night was going to be an exhausting way to make a living if it continued to be full-time.

I said to Alan, my husband and manager, "We have to find a way to make a living where I don't have to show up."

"You mean passive income?" he asked.

"Whatever."

Shortly after that he found the ThighMaster, which went on to become one of the highest-grossing fitness products in America. Passive income and a new career. I began to be introduced on talk shows as a "fitness guru." Once again, I was reinvented. Now I had four careers.

As we reach this incredible transition from the first part of our lives to the second half, it's important to truly examine our patterns of behavior and our ability to grow and adapt to change. Are you in the right frame of mind to be open to new experiences, to challenge how you did things in the past, and to look for ways to improve your life? If not, you are wasting your second chance. Look at people around you and see them continue to create the same cycles over and over again. They aren't reinventing, they are re-creating and not realizing that they are in a rut that isn't working. For example, look at a marriage that may have grown old (as I call it when both parties stop paying attention); divorce is not always the answer. So many people leave one partner and marry the exact same person again. It's important to truly look at reality. Ask yourself, What would I ideally like to have in a partner? Perhaps you need to find a completely different type of person—someone who shares your sensibilities, someone who lives your rhythms, someone who likes to do the same things you do. It's sad, but there is no crime in having grown apart over the years. But first you have to see the part you are playing in this drama called your life. Maybe what needs changing is not your partner, but you.

As I am out and about on the lecture circuit, I often speak to large groups of people about the effects of addictions on the family. I cannot tell you how many times, after one of my lectures, a woman will come up to me and tell me that she has married three alcoholics in a row. She's just had "bad luck in choosing husbands," she usually tells me. But what these women really need to do is understand their patterns of behavior. A different person has more than different hair color and size. The big question is *why* she keeps choosing the same person over and over. It's because this type of person is familiar. She knows who to be and how to be with this type of person.

If I hadn't had the good fortune to find myself in intense therapy in my early twenties, I'm sure I, too, would have married alcoholic after alcoholic. Why? Because I was raised by a violent alcoholic! Being with an alcoholic was familiar and, in its sick way, comfortable. As a child I became codependent before I had ever even heard of the word. Codependency is living someone else's life and not your own. I was owned by my father's moods. If he was happy, I was happy; if he was upset, I was upset. Everything revolved around his moods in our family. The family is as strong as its weakest link. The first question I would ask my mother each morning was "What mood is Daddy in today?" It had nothing to do with my feelings; I needed to know what I needed to do that day to be able to adapt to him.

And adaptable I became. I knew that I liked him during the first couple of hours of his drinking each evening. That's when he thought I was cute and smart and funny. I became his court jester during this period. It's also when I began my life as a "pleaser." I would do anything to keep him happy. What I never understood was that I was not in charge of him. Inevitably, each evening he would pass into the next phase of drunkenness. This was when he got "the means and the hates." He was frightening during this phase. I knew not to say anything to make him volatile. I would readjust my personality to be someone who would fit into his miserable and ugly mood. I would work like a dog around the house. I would polish and clean so he couldn't call me a "lazy asshole." I would make sure he didn't run out of beer. He didn't like it when his can of beer was empty. I figured if I could just keep his beer can from running empty, he might forget about his beloved whiskey chasers. Whiskey made him mean and violent. That was usually when one of us would get hurt, or worse. So many nights the police had to come to our house; so many nights we had to take one of us to the hospital emergency room.

Today this would be called spousal abuse or child abuse; but at that time my father was always able to lie and cajole, convincing the officers that things just "got a little out of hand, ha, ha, ha." They would leave, and then we would experience incredible violence. It was an utterly sad and powerless experience for all of us. I was already too "sick" to understand that the figurative tap dancing we all did trying to please him would not and could not change the outcome of events. Each night was a pattern of the prior night. Hiding the whiskey would just enrage him. If we hadn't been so emotionally controlled by him, we might have realized that the choices he was making for himself were his. And he owned those choices. If he wanted to drink himself to death, that was his choice. I look back and see it was inevitable that beer would never be strong enough to numb the feelings he was trying to push away— that it was merely his "gateway" potion to what he really wanted each night. Inevitably and always, the time would come when he retreated to his whiskey bottle. That was when I knew I had lost the battle for the evening. Now fortified with enough whiskey, he would go after one of us. We never knew who it would be, and we never knew when it was coming. The anticipation was terrifying. I would pray it wouldn't be me, and then I was filled with shame and guilt when it was someone else in the family.

Do you see what was happening to me? I was a little girl with no sense of any right to my own feelings. I had no sense that I had any right to have joy or happiness on my own terms. I could only experience the feelings he was experiencing. As I said, if he was happy, I was happy; if he was upset, I was upset.

Now, you ask, what does this have to do with the subject of this book, which is examining the thrills of aging and making this phase the best your life has ever been? Does it not make sense that if I had not had the opportunity to be "found" in therapy in my early twenties, my patterns of behavior learned from earliest childhood would have seriously affected the choices I made later on as an adult? It is so important to work to undo damage that has been done to you in your life, whether it is caused by poor choices you have made or by circumstances in your life that have created behavioral patterns that do not serve you well.

So when a person comes up to me after a lecture and tells me, "I have married three alcoholics in my life; I guess I'm just unlucky with husbands," I think to myself, You have to go back and find the source of your behavioral patterns. If you have reached this stage of life and have not done this, now is the time. If you haven't been able to put your finger on happiness by this time in your life, then surely something in your past is holding you back. Don't be afraid. Freeing yourself of the shadows of life allows you to be open and receptive to all the good things that want to come your way but have never been able to "get inside" because you have emotional blockages. Going back and correcting the things that need fixing in your emotional self is a gift you give yourself.

Until recently, the general consensus was that women raised the children, dabbled in a career or two, and by the time they reached their mid-fifties it was pretty much over. Today it is quite the contrary. Now, at middle age we have a full half of life left. Thank God we all burned our bras in our twenties to fight for equality and were the first generation that wanted to have relationships that were not like those of our parents. We wanted more and we got it. We wanted to have a real relationship with our kids and husbands. We didn't want to be afraid of our husbands as our mothers were. We wanted our kids to be able to discuss what they were going through without fear. We wanted our kids to know that they were safe with their secrets and that we would help them through the painful times without judgment. We also were the first generation of mothers who had to cope with children using drugs and the sadness and powerlessness of the situation. But we did it and we learned. Through our children, many of us found ourselves in therapy, which became life changing. As with all addictions, those who make it out seem to emerge better and stronger. We learned and adapted, but we have come to another passage. We know our greatest lessons are learned from the dark times in our lives.

Now we are faced with a new challenge. We have half a life left. We have a little money, some even have their houses paid for, our children are raised, and many of us have our darling grandchildren. We are figuring out the hormone mystery. We have cleared every obstacle out of the way, and now we are ready. But for what? To have the most glorious time of our lives! We also have something else, the greatest gift: wisdom. At this time in our lives, we can continue to learn and grow with the advantage of wisdom and make the second half the best that life has ever been.

It takes courage to self-examine. Socrates said, "The unexamined life is not worth living." I have lived my adult life like that. I have chosen to really look at the truth about myself. I don't like what I see sometimes. Sometimes I have to admit things to myself about myself that make me feel ashamed or embarrassed or guilty or remorseful. But to allow myself to know the truth about who I believe I am gives me the tools to change. As I confront these feelings, it becomes painfully clear that I do not want to be owned by any negative choices I have either consciously or subconsciously made. This forces me to start changing myself, and I believe this has been the key to my happiness. Later in this book, I talk more about the importance of reinventing yourself. I have forced myself to do this several times, and because I wasn't afraid to try new things, I have been able to realize incredible dreams for myself after age fifty. These new dreams are based upon recognizing exactly what it is that I now want out of life.

Anyone can do this—it just requires being honest with yourself. So let me ask you once again. You have reached the halfway point. Do you want more of the same, which may already be good; or, if it is not, are you going to take charge of your life and change those things that are not working? It's your life.

As my friend Barry Manilow says: "I believe we are who we choose to be. Nobody is going to come and save you. You've got to save yourself. Nobody is going to give you anything. You've got to go out and fight for it. Nobody knows what you want except you; and nobody will be as sorry as you if you don't get it, so don't give up on your dreams."

Perks of being over forty: No one expects you to run into a burning building.

16

WISDOM

There are clichés about women being competitive with one another, and I think this is true when we are younger because we are full of insecurities and aren't able to take comfort in our relationships with other women. I recall such angst being in the company of mature women when I was younger. These women seemed to have it all together. With young women the competition is mostly about men. It's subliminal, for if women really thought about it, we would realize how ridiculous this unconscious vying for attention truly is. As we age, we realize the importance of friendship with other women. We seem to enjoy comparing wrinkles and laughing about it—kind of a "misery loves company."

It seems as though one morning you wake up and your skin is like an ill-fitting suit. What can you do? There is no plastic surgeon who can pick up the slack on your overall body. Face lifts, collagen, and Botox are all temporary Band-Aids that can indeed make you look better. Collagen can fill in lines on the face, Botox can temporarily lift eyebrows, foreheads, the eye area, and even zap the veins in your neck to appear less obvious. But the skin continues to age and sag. Skin deterioration is helped tremendously by replacing lost hormones, but gravity does exist and some things are going to happen no matter what you do.

This is where girlfriends come into play. It's comforting to be able to share the startling effects of aging with a good friend. It creates a bond of loyalty and trust, which over time allows you to open up to one another without judgment. Isn't it great how, with age, we acquire the wisdom to see that women are our friends, not our competitors? Just think what we would have been like if we'd had this kind of confidence and devil-may-care attitude when we were younger. As we approach middle age, we gain a whole new perspective on who we are in the world. We may not be the youngest, hottest babes in the room anymore, but what we have lost in this area we have gained in wisdom and confidence. This is a great trade-off. By this age it is necessary to get over being the prettiest, curviest, or most attractive. Instead, be the most fabulous, interesting, intelligent, charming, and funny woman in the room. That's where the real sexiness clicks in. Once you figure this out, you'll start having more fun than ever before.

Recently, while in New York, I had lunch at a hip, trendy restaurant with a female editor in chief of a very popular magazine. I'd guess she is either in her late fifties or early sixties, but it doesn't matter because she looks great for any age. She is a mother, a grandmother, happily married, and successful in her business. She wore her thick, naturally silver hair at a fabulous shoulder length, had on a beautiful business suit, a little makeup, and confidence galore. Ours was a fabulous table at which to be seated because she held court to some of the most exciting, interesting, and successful men in the entertainment and journalism world. One by one they came to our table to talk with her. She looked great, but it was her confidence that made her stunning. Because of this great self-assuredness, she was sexy. The men joked with her, flirted with her, wanted to do business with her, were not threatened by her, and respected her and her accomplishments. Her sexy femininity attracted them like a magnet. She was in tune with herself, her age, her success, and her attractiveness, and she radiated a wisdom about who she was and what she wanted out of life that was very appealing.

This is how it works for the woman who is comfortable with herself and her age. For the first time in your life, everyone in the room is now taking you seriously. You have reached an age where you have formed your opinions. They are not the opinions of others; instead, at this age you have enough perspective to have formed your own ideas. You carry your own at any dinner party. People who in your younger years dismissed your theories are now interested in your point of view. It's fantastic. People who once would have intimidated you are now seen by you as just "people." As you get older, you realize that there are no big shots. I've watched the most powerful be knocked down. Everyone is vulnerable. Wisdom allows you to realize that.

You finally understand that money does not define a person; only integrity and decency matter. There are wealthy people who are amazing, but it is never about their wealth. It's about who they are and what they think and feel. It's about being caring and compassionate. This is an amazing time of life, but only if you have done the work that leads up to it. There is no room for dysfunction at this age. It's time to get over it, and that requires taking a good look at yourself. Those things from your past or your childhood must stop running your life. If you haven't been able to face the demons of your past, what are you waiting for? That alcoholic father is going to win if you are still being run by the voices within you that resonate the mocking and ridicule he used to dish out. It's time to look at the situation from another angle: What was his need to badger you so? Was it his way of coping with his own sense of inadequacy?

In my life, I allowed my father to convince me that I was "stupid, hopeless, worthless, nothin', and a big zero," just as he had always said to me in his drunken rages. It never dawned on me as a child that this was really what he thought about himself. It never dawned on me that this was his tactic to keep me under his control. As long as I was emotionally handicapped by his badgering, I wouldn't leave him, and that was what he wanted. Without us, he knew he would eventually have to look at the reality of what he had done with his life. That picture of himself was too painful, so he kept himself anesthetized with booze, and the liquor gave him the emotional mustering to hold us in his reign of terror.

The greatest thing I ever did for myself was get professional help. It was through therapy that I was finally able to realize that what happened to me as a child was not my fault. That was revelatory because I had always assumed I had been born bad. Why would I think anything else when I had been told over and over since infancy that I was stupid and hopeless? As adults we forget the impact we have on children. To understand the world from a child's point of view, lie on the floor and look up. Look at how big we appear to be. Children are shaped by those in charge of raising them; everything we are, good and bad, is a result of the input of those who raised us. As adults, it is our job to keep the good parts of us and correct those things in our person that need fixing. If those corrections are not made, the negative influences of our past win. At this point it's your fault.

You have the opportunity in life to overcome and make changes, to shape yourself into the person you want to be. Few of us realize that we are in control of our lives. We must decide what we want from life and then go after it. It takes shaping and tending, much like a beautiful garden. The garden may start out as a barren patch of scruffy earth, but with toil and lots of work it turns into a thing of beauty and joy. Life works the same way. If you haven't started doing the work at this point, then you have a lot of catching up to do, but it's not impossible. It will require total honesty on your part. You have to really look at why you haven't wanted to face the reality of who you have become. It is usually fear and emotional pain that drive us. It's also agitating to dig up those things you'd rather forget from your past, but the fact that you don't want to face them reveals that the issue is still bringing you pain. Take the chance. Face the pain. It will be the most important thing you have ever done for yourself, as important as balancing your hormones.

You cannot imagine how much these old issues hold you down. Coming to terms and then to true forgiveness releases that part of you that has never had a chance to develop because you have been so busy, so clever and cunning, in avoiding the realities. Holding on to old pain can make you sick. It is a proven fact that stress is a major factor in causing disease. You cannot escape from old issues; you can only bury them—but they don't go away. Pay attention to the things in life that make you emotional. What makes you cry? What triggers your emotions? These emotions are you talking to yourself. This is you trying to release old pain. Pay attention to what triggers your feelings, because feelings are our truth. In fact, the smartest part of us is our feelings. They never lie.

If you find yourself crying, figure out what released the flood of emotions. I have a friend who cries every time someone in the family leaves for a trip. She still aches from losing her mother at a young age. Her mother went into the hospital and never came out, so that has left her with abandonment issues. At some point in her life, she will have to do the work to go back and relive the painful time in her childhood when she lost the most important person in the world to her. It will be upsetting. Perhaps she will discover hidden anger. At that time, in order to protect them, children were never told what was truly going on. Maybe she is still angry about not being properly informed of the reason her mother left and not being able to say good-bye in the way she would have wanted.

Maybe the child in her has anger that her mother left her. This has nothing to do with the fact that her mother had no choice; we are talking about the pain of that moment in her childhood, which remains hidden inside her with a child's intensity. You grow up, but the pain does not. The things we don't want to face don't mature. We mature, but the pain is the pain of our child self, pure and without logic or adult understanding. It is the leftover stuff from our past that keeps us from being all that we can be. If this resonates in any way with you, find yourself a group or a good therapist and get it out of you. You can't imagine how freeing it is.

People always comment that I seem so happy, and it's because I am. You know why . . . because I got to the bottom of it. All the books I have written have mostly been about trying to find out why I am the way I am and what I can do to change those things about myself that are in my way. My feelings about my alcoholic father kept me in a chokehold all of my life. My insecurity over-whelmed my life. I never felt I was good enough for anything. After years of searching, I was finally able to crawl out from under these feelings and see the light. Once I could see, life became easier, more enjoyable, more successful, sexier! Had I not done the work, I don't know where I would be today. There is not a room I walk into where I don't feel I belong. The agitation, the sadness, and the anger I felt during my years of therapy seem so insignificant now. Doing the work was worth it. It changed me and allowed me to become a person I enjoy being.

Once you have taken the big step to make the necessary correc-tions within yourself, you are prepared to receive your new wis-dom. When your thinking is not clouded with negatives and old unresolved issues, the wise part of you takes over. Wisdom is your ability to assess situations. Wise people "get it." Wise people don't overreact. Wise people listen to all sides and make informed deci-sions. Wise people are easy to be around because you know you are going to be treated fairly. There is a sense of balance and seren-ity associated with wisdom. You feel and appear peaceful (as long as your hormones are balanced).

Wisdom gives you an inner sense that you can handle any situa-tion. This is no small thing. Acquired wisdom allows you to know that you can handle whatever curve is thrown your way. Wisdom leaves the girl behind, and the woman who emerges is so much more attractive. So much energy is spent at this age trying to cap-ture lost youth, instead of putting emphasis and focus on the new passages. It is the calm of this age that makes you attractive. Calm is cool. Cool is sexy. Wisdom rocks!

Perks of being over forty:
There is nothing else to learn the hard way.

17

TAKING CHARGE OF YOUR LIFE

Middle age really is a wonderful opportunity to reinvent yourself. I talked about the importance of reinvention a bit in chapter 15 and how we need to reinvent ourselves throughout our whole lives. Don't despair—it's never too late to do other things with your life, and now is the best time to be open to new opportunities. Your kids are out of the house, your husband may be slowing down in his career. Now it's time to ask yourself what passions you have always had. It is the best time possible to fulfill dreams or create new ones. I have found that it has been helpful in my life, when trying to figure out what my dreams are, to ask myself what it was that I did when I was a child that totally engaged me. In what activities did I lose myself? Ask yourself the same question: What were the activities that engaged you so deeply that time passed without noticing? These activities are clues to remembering what it is that you love to do and think about.

Maturity is remembering the revelation that all along we have been trying to get back to where we started. I used to play house. Not surprisingly, I am now heavily involved with creating a home-wares division on Home Shopping Network (HSN), including appliances, kitchenware, and bedding. In addition, I recently contracted with my publisher to write a book on lifestyle. My hugely successful Somersize line of books came out of my love of cooking, not just a desire to lose weight. I have always loved being in the kitchen, and I became consumed with trying to find delicious dishes that would keep me and my family healthy. It's essential to continue redefining your life from passage to passage. If I hadn't done this, I might be one of those "has-beens" or features on one of those "whatever happened to" shows on television.

I realize that not everyone has the opportunity to sell satin bedding, housewares, and jewelry on television, but look realistically at what it is that you can do within the arena of your interests. The redefining of my life seems to have no connection with the passage that preceded it, yet there is a thread of continuity. Each new endeavor has to do with growth and strength and a yearning to find out who I am and what makes me tick. I'm not ready to sit by the fire and stare. One day that will be nice, but right now I have too much energy and excitement. In ways I feel younger now than ever before, because I have nothing to prove to anyone, not even to myself. I am now driven by my interests.

You can do this, too. I go to many farmers' markets to buy fresh produce, and I see women of all ages setting up little boutique stands and selling wonderful items that they have made themselves. It is very empowering as a woman to make your own money. Even if it's money to spend just on yourself or the house, it puts you in control and allows you the freedom to make choices for yourself. We still live in a world where men are better paid and have better opportunities than women. But things are changing. By being proactive about your life and finances, not only are you making it easier for women of the next generation, but you are also teaching your children about the resiliency and creativity of women.

So many of the woman I talked with in this book referred to this incredible burst of energy, and I believe it's because for the first time they realize they are finally in control of their own lives and can pursue them in any way they'd like. When you are turned on by life, you are sexy. Tune in to your feelings: is there an inner calling you've put on hold for so long that you have forgotten about it? When my mother died, I came across some beautiful watercolor drawings that she had done when she attended the Lux School of

Design in San Francisco. I can remember her speaking about Lux, but my father would always make fun of her and put her down. Because of his reaction, we children would join in what I now realize was ridicule. But when my sister and brother and I were cleaning out her house after her death, I cried when I saw those drawings. They were good, really good. In fact, I now have them beautifully framed and kept in one of her favorite guestrooms in my home. I go to that room often to look at them. They make me feel happy and sad simultaneously.

Women of my mother's age put aside their dreams to raise their families. That's the way it used to be. Women of my mother's generation were not supposed to "have it all," and I'm sure frustration was inherent in that role. Today most women have found a way to have it all, but few have found balance. We are still learning how to juggle gracefully. My mother was angry and bitter for many years because of my father's violent alcoholism, but after seeing these drawings, I now believe that some of that frustration was also a result of not being able to express herself creatively. She was always so supportive of my endeavors, I'm sure through me she was able to fulfill some of her dreams. But the lesson is clear: Life is short, and if you don't get out of it what you want, it's your loss! It's a waste of time to sit around talking about how unfair things are. No one's future turns out the way it was expected to. Life changes for everyone, and it's important to adjust and find another way—that's true creativity.

As we get older, achievement is still important, but we are driven more by personal fulfillment than by what others think. That's why I find this age to be so exciting. I finally feel it's my time. I am now the captain of my ship. It's a waste of time to care what others think. If you do, you are owned by them. Instead, we have to ask what we can do each day to fulfill our dreams. It's exciting to change your life. But change brings risk, and it does get harder as we get older because we become set in our ways. It's frightening to start all over, but change brings a new burst of energy. At middle age, my sister and her husband lost their entire fortune. She had never worked, and after a period of grief and mourning, she rolled up her sleeves and got her real estate license. It wasn't easy. She began by knocking on doors and going from house to house to get listings. She encountered many of the people with whom she used to attend all the fancy parties. She held her head up high, and today she is one of the leading real estate salespeople in the country. She took the risk, put aside her fear, and changed her life. Whenever I am having a bad day, I always call my sister because I know just hearing the excitement in her voice will cheer me up.

These are the kinds of things we can do as women to grow and move forward. Women today are taking more risks because tomorrow appears hopeful. Women have made tremendous progress; the doors of opportunity have opened wider than ever before. We are being heard, and we have rights, although we still have to fight for them, but that is part of the challenge and excitement. There are many women today who are opening their own businesses. Women are redefining the concept of "old." Women in their fifties and sixties are looking hot. Women are achieving great things in areas formerly closed to them. Madeleine Albright became secretary of state at the age of fifty-nine! Women are running studios and corporations; they are exercising, they are proactive about their health, they are having affairs with younger and younger men. Frankly, for me, I enjoy the fact that my husband is ten years older; this way I always get to be the young one. But my girlfriends with young boyfriends seem pretty darned happy, and I have to say there is a glow to their skin.

We women of this generation are exceptional beings. We have rewritten the rules. We are the first generation of women to use therapy as a tool for being happier people. We didn't want to have relationships like those of our parents. We didn't want to have a divide between us and our children, we wanted to talk to them; we wanted them to be comfortable coming to us with any problem. That has made for true intimacy with our children and our spouses. This is a remarkable breakthrough. And we are now experiencing the payoff. Our children are our best friends. There is no one I would rather be with than my son, Bruce, and his family. Bruce is my confidant and I am his. There is no subject too uncomfortable; we are able to talk about anything. Because of this I never feel excluded from his life, nor he from mine. Therapy allowed me to be this way. I certainly didn't learn this in my parents' home. My mother had one personality when she was with us and another when my father was around. If he walked into the room, we stopped talking. When my mother was with her friends, she was relaxed and comfortable; when my father was with her, she sat stiff and uncomfortable.

Therapy allows you to understand the buried anxieties and rages. You can't grow and be able to change if you don't recognize what has made you angry for so long. If you are to have a long and happy life, you have to get to the bottom of all buried pain so you can understand it, forgive, and move forward. Once it is understood, you can let it go and find forgiveness not only for those who caused you pain, but also for the part you played in the drama of your life. If you didn't have a perfect relationship with either or both of your parents, do the work and then get over it. You are an adult now, and you don't need your mommy or daddy to have a happy life. If you didn't "get" what you wanted or thought you wanted, do the work to discover what that was (usually it's love) and then find that love in your own life. Get rid of old jealousies and resentments. If you don't, these emotions will pull you down. You will be the loser. Stay clear of people who are jealous of you. They too will pull you down. Envy is something you aspire to, jealousy is not wanting others to have what they have. Envy is a positive emotion, as in "I want to be like you"; jealousy is a negative emotion, as in "I don't want you to have what you have." Nothing good comes from jealousy. It's destructive, mean-spirited, and petty. Run, don't walk, away from it.

I know a middle-aged man who has everything going for him—great looks, great physique, intelligence, creativity, humor, and energy—except he is jealous of everyone. He is constantly looking over his shoulder and at who is ahead of him, and he wonders why he can't get his life on track. His jealousy is holding him back. It's impossible for him to be all that he can be because so much of his time is wasted on not wanting others to have what they have.

You have worked too hard your whole life to get mired now in petty emotions like jealousy. These negative emotions will hold you back and prevent you from realizing your dreams. You have to be a self-starter. You have got to figure out what you want from this next phase of your life and then decide how to get it. An optimist sees opportunity in every difficulty, and a pessimist sees difficulty in every opportunity. Be an optimist. Look at everything that has happened to you, good and bad, as an opportunity to grow and learn spiritually and emotionally. Turn your lemons into lemonade. Make your greatest problems your greatest opportunity. Take charge of your life and make it exactly what you want it to be. We all have made mistakes, and we will continue to do so, but at this age we realize it's the problems and mistakes that are our greatest opportunities, if we choose to look at them that way. We learn from our past, but the challenge is to not repeat patterns of behavior that are not serving us well.

Perks of being over forty:
Your husband jokes that instead of
buying a woodstove, he is using you
to heat the family room this winter.
Rather than just saying you are
not amused, you shoot him.

18

STAYING COOL

The surest way to guess somebody's age is by their "cool" factor. Staying cool is being comfortable in your skin. It's about liking your age. I remember listening to an interview with Steve Allen one day, and the interviewer said, "You were always one of the really cool guys." And Steve Allen replied, "If you're cool, you're always cool. Just because I'm an old guy now doesn't mean I'm not cool anymore." He was right: just because you get older doesn't mean you suddenly change your take on things. For instance, how old is Jack Nicholson? You never really think about his age, do you? It's because Jack is just a cool guy. So it doesn't matter if he's fifty, eighty, or one hundred, he's still this sexy, impish, mischievous guy. He seems as if he'd be fun to hang around with, and all because he's cool!

Frank Sinatra was cool. It was never about his age. We didn't care if he was getting older; if fact, as he got older he seemed to get sexier. It's because he always stayed cool. He was the type of guy you could still fantasize about sleeping with even when he was eighty years old. What about Sting or Rod Stewart? They're cool guys because they have created their own style and don't care what people think. They have the right to express themselves in any way they want. You never think about their age; they are just these two sexy guys.

"Cool" is ageless. It's your take on things. It's about not being judgmental. It's about acceptance. If your girlfriend has decided to dye her hair pink and pierce her nose or other body parts, you are okay with it because that's the way she has decided to decorate herself. Don't we earn the right to be, dress, pierce, or adorn ourselves in any way we want? It really doesn't matter how it ends up looking, it's all about expressing ourselves in any way we want because we have earned the right to be whoever we choose to be. It's our life. We are finally in control of ourselves at this age. We've spent a lifetime trying to do what's right and appropriate, and now we can stop being governed by what the rest of the community is doing or what the magazines tell us we should be doing or how we should be dressing. The women who write those articles are all in their twenties anyway.

I think by now we know what's best for us without a twenty-year-old advising us, yet being cool is about being open to what a twenty-year-old has to say, or anyone of any age, for that matter. Some twenty-year-olds are very wise and old souls, and it might just be that they are telling us exactly what we need to hear at that moment. Always be open to the messages, because you never know where they might be coming from. Some of my greatest messages have come from the mouths of my grandchildren.

When I was a child, I always heard that at a certain age (forty was the cutoff), a woman should cut her hair short. All my life I have had long hair; I find it the most versatile. I can braid it, put it on top of my head, wear a ponytail, or style it straight or curly. With long hair I have options. Today it's not about what's appropriate, it's about what looks best, without looking desperate. It's a matter of taste. You have to look in the mirror and decide what looks best. This is where your good taste and wisdom come in. If you are more comfortable with your hair long, then by all means that's how you should wear it. It's up to you to know if it looks great or stupid. Wearing clothes that make you look desperate makes you look stupid. You have to know who you are. What's right for Cher (one of the really cool chicks) may or may not be right for you. Personally, I wouldn't look good in any of her getups. A bare midriff is not my style, but you have to admit, Cher looks great all the time, always has, probably always will. She's always been cool. It's not forced; it's her personal style and expression. That's the goal. Wear what you feel comfortable wearing and be who you want to be.

Now is the time to step out of the box. Buy yourself a black leather skirt if that is something you would feel comfortable in. Recently, I saw Maria Shriver wearing a long black leather skirt, black stiletto boots, a black turtleneck sweater, and a strand of pearls. She looked great. It was her personal style. It was hip, edgy, not desperate; yet she still maintained a ladylike demeanor, because that is who she is. She is someone who is comfortable in her own skin. She's a great mother, has a fabulous marriage and a career of her own invention. She seems to work when it is convenient for her. With four children and as wife of the governor she obviously has taken the time to invent her life so she can have it all.

We look at someone like Maria Shriver and think she was born with a silver spoon in her mouth. Granted, she was born into privilege; but Maria had a lot of disadvantages to overcome. Because she was a Kennedy, the pressure to succeed was enormous. No other member of her family had ever ventured into television. I'm sure there was disapproval within the family, but Maria started at the bottom and worked her way up. I remember in the early eighties, I used to run into her in the back rooms of television studios doing intern work, while I was waiting to go on *The Charlie Rose Show*. She had determination and a desire to have it all. We've seen her hosting the *Today* show while pregnant, then we'll spot her at a premiere with her husband, Arnold Schwarzenegger, looking very fancy, then we'll see a candid shot of her walking around Santa Monica without makeup looking very unglamorous, pushing a baby carriage. She's cool because she doesn't care what anyone thinks of her. She's doing it her way, dressing her way, having her marriage her way, establishing a career her way.

A very important aspect of aging is taking a good look at yourself and assessing your look. The surest way to date yourself is by wearing the same makeup you wore in your twenties or thirties.

Most of us do that. Imagine how I would look if I were still wearing the makeup that served me so well when I was playing Chrissy Snow on *Three's Company*. I wore thick black eyeliner all the way around the eye, lots of white highlight under the eye, cotton candy pink blush in big pink rounds on my cheeks, and big pink glossy lips. Top that with pure white-blond hair pulled into two ponytails on either side of my head, and you have my look of the 1980s. It was real cute then, but today, at fifty-six, I would look quite desperate . . . kind of like *Whatever Happened to Baby Jane*.

I remember the day I looked in the mirror and realized that that look of the eighties was no longer serving me well. It had outlived its purpose. Instead of looking cute and perky, I looked old and overly made-up. Suddenly, what once worked now looked unattractive. I scrubbed my face and made the decision to change the color of my hair. White-blond hair is great when you are in your twenties, but in my early forties it drained me of my color and forced me to wear a lot of makeup to fill in the color. I changed my hair to a more natural blond with gold highlights and my makeup to softer, more natural colors. It was an amazing transformation for me. Suddenly people were telling me I looked younger, softer, prettier.

We need to change and update our looks from passage to passage. It says something about ourselves. It says that we are not stuck in a time warp, that we are not holding on to what was, or to "the good old days." Change looks fresh and shows forward motion. If you think you've lost all that was remarkable and valuable about your youth, then you really have to think about why that time in your life was better for you than now. But here's the point: Youth is gone. Today is what is important, so examine why "today" is not bringing you contentment and satisfaction.

Perks of being over forty: You enjoy
hearing about other people's operations.

19

MAUREEN: A SIXTY-THREE-YEAR-OLD EXPERIENCE

Maureen is my sister, sixty-three years old and a real estate super-salesperson. Like me, she is a breast cancer survivor and is on natural bioidentical hormone replacement therapy. As you will read in this chapter, she is enjoying her life to the fullest. She does not want to turn back the clock. Her energy, vitality, and libido are operating at optimum. In speaking to her, I kept trying to find any negatives associated with taking natural bioidentical hormones, but I wasn't able to pull any out of her. She even went so far as to say that she thinks the quality of her life is so spectacular that even if bioidentical hormones were to shorten her life, it would be worth it. That's quite an endorsement.

You've heard from me and my fifty-year-old (ish) point of view relative to replacing lost hormones with real hormones, but listen to my sister talk about hormones from her perspective as a sixty-three-year-old. Maureen is honest to a fault and has graciously shared her point of view.

Before I took bioidentical hormones, I felt dead. The lights were out, my spirit felt dead. I remember wishing a lot, for anything . . . a windfall, winning the lottery, getting back what I had lost. It was a terrible time in my life. I think menopause is a very difficult time for women because a lot of things are going on. For instance, you've had your animals for a long time and they start dying around this age. It's sad and hard. Both my dogs died, my birds died, I lost both of my houses because of the real estate crash of the 1980s, so we lost all our money. For the first time in my life, I realized I had to get a job, but how do you get into the workforce at this age after never having been in the workforce to begin with? I was scared and intimidated, and on top of all of this I had no hormones.

I had no libido. Nothing. I slept in the fetal position for three years, and I wouldn't let my husband touch me. I felt like the frozen chicken in the freezer, packed real tight with clamps on my legs holding them together. Believe me, I made sure that no one reaching in there to get at that package was going to find anything. I was fifty-two then and kept thinking, This can't be happening to me. I was never a complainer. I never complained about my period or cramps. I would be annoyed at the women who complained, and I would think, Oh, grow up, or, Get over it, as I listened to them.

Then I got breast cancer, so I took myself off the prescribed drug hormones I was taking. I went without them for three years. Evidently, one night I was acting so badly that the next day a girlfriend took me out to lunch and put a patch (drug hormones) on me. I realized my mood had been awful, and I did feel some relief from the patch. But then I started gaining weight. I just blew up. I gained so much weight when I started on the patch that I went off them also.

My sexless, angry, depressed life went on like this until I felt that I'd rather not be alive anymore. My days were not bringing me any joy, and I am a happy person by nature. People have always told me how great it is to be around me because I am so "up," but not anymore. I didn't even recognize myself. Everything made me angry, and I was ready to blame my husband at every turn. (No wonder men leave their wives at this age.)

I went to see Dr. Schwarzbein because my sister, Suzanne, seemed to be so pleased with her progress. After all, she had breast cancer also and was enjoying her life on a hormonal basis, so I decided I'd give it a try. As soon as I was on real bioidentical hormones, I was a different girl. Suddenly I couldn't get enough sex. I was in my prime again, and I was actually wearing out my husband (well, maybe not). I thought, Wow, this is fantastic. Yippee! An "E" ticket. But I soon realized there is more to it than getting your sex drive back (although I must say this alone makes all the rest you have to go through more tolerable).

It's not been easy to find balance. On real hormones I also gained weight. This was depressing. I went up to 150 pounds. My normal weight is 127. My metabolism was so out of whack from the drug hormones and the carbohydrates I had been eating. At the time we were struggling financially, so we went out to dinner a lot because of our work overload, and I had started eating bread. It was inexpensive, and it was always sitting on the table while we waited for our dinner, and it would fill me up so we didn't have to spend so much money. All these carbohydrates threw my hormone levels further out of whack, and now I was insulin resistant, and I didn't even know what that was. All I knew was that I had these two "hams" on either side of my hips, right at the top below your waist, where it makes everything you wear look terrible, and for the first time in my life I had a big ass. The weight made me feel terrible about myself, but the hormones were giving me a renewed zest about life. I had a big ole butt, but my husband and I were having nightly romps of great sex.

My doctor told me that hormonal balance takes patience. I had damaged my metabolism from years of incorrect eating, plus the damage done earlier in my life when I was drinking alcohol (I have been sober for twenty-five years); also, all that time without taking any kind of hormone replacement had left me at zero. I had no hormones. No wonder I felt dead. No wonder I had no will to live. No wonder I was taking it all out on my dear husband. Dr. Schwarzbein said that it would take a few years for everything to find its balance and that eventually the weight would come off, but I had to eat properly to heal my damaged metabolism. Initially, she said, this food would put on weight while it was doing its good work of rebuilding. We also found out that I had plaque in my arteries and I had seriously high blood pressure. All the things you hear about old people were happening to me. But in spite of all of this information, the real hormones were giving me a renewed zest.

I was starting a new career, I was recovering from the shock of having had breast cancer, I was gaining weight, but I was still happier than I had been in a long time, and it had to be because of the hormones. I could feel myself getting stronger, and because of this I made a commitment to myself to become my doctor's best patient. I decided to approach this in the same way I had tackled my alcoholism. I was going to do everything she said and really give this a try. I realized I couldn't do this thing half-assed. The struggle was softened, however, because of the real hormone replacement.

I remembered a story that my mother used to read to me as a child, about "the little train that could," so I used that as a metaphor—"I think I can, I think I can." I started lifting weights, all the while saying to myself, "I can do this." I began meditating and started reading a lot of spiritual books that allowed me to see this not as a time of despair, but as an opportunity to grow and change. I knew I needed to change my life, and these books were giving me the tools to do so. At times I still wanted to hide in the freezer like that chicken, and I didn't want to face my children, but I hung in and continued to do the work physically and emotionally.

It's been hard, that's for sure, but it's becoming worth it. There is no magic pill. Real hormones definitely are the answer, but you've got to be willing to do the work that accompanies this balance. You can't think, now that you are replacing your lost hormones with real hormones, that this is the beginning and the end. If you continue to eat sugar (I ate mine in the form of carbohydrates), you will keep getting fat. The real hormones work by improving your overall well-being; but if you are eating badly, all that sugar is going to interfere with your body's ability to keep your hormones balanced.

Taking real hormones has made me healthier in every way. I realize that if I want a sex life this satisfying, I have to obey the rules. I have to be rigorously honest with myself and my doctors. You can't lie to your doctors; it defeats the purpose. You have to tell them if you are sneaking sugar, otherwise they won't be able to help you properly. They aren't going to sit there and tell you that you are a liar. It's not up to them. If you want to get better, you have to be accountable to yourself. Just as I approached alcoholism, I now do this "one day at a time." If that gets too difficult, I do it one hour at a time or one moment at a time. I want this to work. But I am driving that little train.

Today I am feeling great. My weight is 129. I still have a few more pounds to get rid of. It's taken me four years. That's a lot of patience. But I am eating fantastic meals. Because of my high blood pressure and the fact that I am still insulin resistant to a small degree, I am also watching my fat intake until my levels are acceptable. I visualize that all this great food I am eating is slowly cleaning out my arteries. When my insulin levels are normal, and my blood pressure is normal, and I drive away the plaque through visualization and a healthy lifestyle and diet, I get to incorporate real fats again with more frequency. I do love butter and cream.

I believe I will stay on real hormones forever. If I die because of it (which I don't think will happen), it will have been worth it. I can't describe the well-being you get from replacing lost hormones with the real ones. Frankly, life wasn't worth living the other way.

I have taken those kinds of chances to afford me a better quality of life. I took birth control pills for a long time (almost two decades). I am very fertile, and after having four children, three of them in three successive years, I found that birth control pills gave me a better quality of life at that time. I didn't have to say no to my husband, and it was the one time of the day just for us. With four kids, there is not much time in the day for meaningful conversation. I feel the same way about hormone replacement. I am willing to take the risk. I am really living these days; before I started on real hormones, I felt like the walking dead.

I am accountable for my health. I realized the power we have within when I went through breast cancer. I worked with a healer who truly taught me that we were body, mind, and spirit. This whole passage of life is completely up to me. I absolutely have to be honest with my doctors and the people who are helping me through this period, and keep them informed so they can do their best work. It's stupid to BS your doctors. I have made my choices. It's not going to be anyone's fault, regardless of the outcome. I am not mad at the medical profession. Doctors today are so busy that it is almost impossible for them to keep up with recent studies. Therefore, it is up to me. I am accountable for my health, my spirit, my body. I am accountable for myself in the financial world; because of that I have a coach I work with once a week to improve my business and my relationships with my working team, who happen to be my family.

I am grateful for the new integrated medicine. It's truly interactive, and there is a new respect between doctor and patient in terms of getting to the bottom of what ails you. No longer is medicine a Band-Aid to slap on till the symptoms clear up. Now we are able to go deeper—holistic, if you will—to find out not only what it is, but also what caused it.

When my hormones are balanced, I am turned on about practically everything. I feel great about everything. I love my age. It's a good age. When I meet my contemporaries, I notice that many of them are really getting old. I know the difference between them and me is hormones. I think the big difference is that I have sex regularly. I talk about it. I love it. I never hear any of my girlfriends talking about it. In fact, in your sixties, there is a lot of laughter about the fact that you are not having sex anymore.

I think for me the big difference is sex, not only having sex, but also wanting it. It's a great time of life—there are no interruptions, the kids are gone, there is no right or wrong, just pleasure.

To other women my age who haven't got a handle on things, I would like to say: Take yourself on—be accountable. Find out who you are in every way, and find out all that you can be. Be sure to take care of yourself. Go to the doctor. Try a new one. Switch around. When you hear about a doctor who has a new approach, get an appointment and find out what he or she is up to. Get X-rays, take the latest tests. Take hold of your life. When you start menopause, everything is going to change. This passage requires absolute, rigorous honesty and lots of work, but take it from me, I feel enthusiastic about absolutely everything.

I owe my life to these hormones. Without them I felt and behaved badly. Am I ever glad to leave that part of me behind.

"Old" is when . . . a sexy babe
catches your man's fancy and his pacemaker
opens the garage door.

20

RELATIONSHIPS

Hormones are a wonderful component of who we are. They give us life and balance. They make our systems work properly; they make our skin glow, our hair shiny and healthy, our nails strong; and they radiate on the outside the balance within. But hormones can also be responsible for conflict that we have with our partners. Sometimes what seems real, like a relationship problem, might be caused by a chemical imbalance. Think PMS! Remember that time of the month when your chemicals were wonky and you found yourself wondering what ever attracted you to your husband in the first place? Then as soon as you were back in balance, the angry and negative thoughts from a few days ago seemed laughable? Menopause can make you feel like that all the time, so it seems real that your husband is a jerk. I wonder how many marriages break up because of menopause? I wonder how many families could have remained intact if there had been a better understanding of the chemical imbalance that accompanies menopause? It is so important to understand this passage. Everything can be brought into balance through a blood test and a qualified endocrinologist or doctor "in the know."

So don't make any rash decisions or accusations until you have found balance. But if after achieving this balance you still are not happy with your mate and the life you are living, then you can make real decisions for yourself that are not the result of hormonal imbalance. Take a good, hard look at your life. Is your partner boring you? Remember, you have another whole half of your life to spend with this person. Is it worth it? Have the two of you forgotten to notice each other over the years? Is life without your kids empty and void? Do you hate your work? Is sex a distant memory? Do you pine over the body you once had? Have you given up on joy? If your answer is yes to any one of these, it's time to do some emotional work.

Here's the thing: you can change every one of these components, but you are going to have to commit to some hard work. If that puts you off, then you have to ask yourself why you are not willing to put out the effort to change yourself and your life. I agree it's no easy task to revive a marriage that has lost its glow. It's even harder to admit that you no longer have any interest in trying to put the glow back into your marriage. If that is so, it requires a huge change on your part. Divorce could change your financial situation, you might have to go to work for the first time in your life, it might make you feel frightened, and with good reason—but look at the alternative. If you are going to live for another fifty years (and you are, barring some kind of accident), is it worth it to give the second half to a situation that is hopeless or, worse, loveless?

Don't live a loveless life. To be trapped in a situation that has no love is to feel dead inside. You will never find your inner glow living a loveless life. Perhaps you can learn to enjoy your partner as a friend or companion, someone you like to take drives with or to share a home with; but you have to acknowledge this new way of thinking to yourself so you can turn the page and realize that what you once had together no longer exists—it's dead. Your relationship can be reshaped to be something other than what it once was. This is workable, because this person is obviously someone who has qualities that are important to you. How can this relationship be salvaged? By understanding that now it will be on different terms that the two of you find mutually agreeable. In other words, the two of you need to agree to new terms of living together. If your husband (or wife) still interests you as a person with whom sharing a house and occasional social events is enough, then that can bring you happiness.

It is important to address the changes in your relationship to avoid becoming bitter and angry because things are no longer the way they were. In a scenario like this, it is important to establish a life of your own. Make friends of your own, plan lunches and dinners without your mate. Have your own life, but accept the new arrangement responsibly. You want him, but not the way you once wanted him. Accept that this arrangement works both ways. He will want to hang out with his own friends, have lunches and dinners also. You can't be angry with him for having a life without you, because this is what you have both chosen.

I am grateful to be very happily married, so this scenario would not work with my marriage, but for some couples this is a way of holding on to all that the two of them have created. It is easier on your grown kids, your family is whole, and the two of you are no longer frustrated, angry, and bitter. When you do share an evening together or an occasional sexual romp, you can enjoy each other without all the residual resentment that used to ruin your evenings. Who knows, maybe this way you will fall in love with each other all over again. Maybe when the two of you rearrange your present life, each of you might notice how cool your partner has become. But don't count on it, or you will have expectations that could set you up for disappointment.

No matter what path you take with your partner, this is your chance to have the life you want. Take responsibility for your life and your relationships and how they have turned out. And if you don't like what you see, then start doing the work necessary to create the life you want.

"Old" is when . . . your friends
compliment you on your new alligator
shoes and you're barefoot.

21

MAKING SENSE OF IT

In comparing the points of view of women taking natural bioidentical hormones with those of women who are not, it's apparent to me that the ones who are replacing their lost hormones with real hormones are enjoying the best quality of life. Maureen, my sister, went so far as to say that even if taking bioidentical HRT shortened her life, it will have been worth it because of the difference it's made in how much she enjoys each day.

Life is better on real hormones. Without them we start slowly to fade away. At one time we expected to be like this as we got older, but today it doesn't have to happen. Bioidentical hormone replacement allows you to enjoy a fabulous quality of life, filled with energy and the zest for living. Your health will be better, too, because taking bioidentical hormones helps prevent the onset of the diseases of aging.

My sister experienced terrible mood swings when she first entered menopause. It was a terrible time for both of us, because neither of us knew what was going on. She went on drug hormones and her mood got better, but then things started going wrong metabolically. She started gaining weight, and then because of breast cancer she stopped taking the drug hormones, so her hormone levels zeroed out.

During the three years without hormones she became a person I didn't recognize. She spoke in a flat voice, her enthusiasm was gone, and she said things like "I feel dead." The sister I grew up with, the sister I aspired to be when I was growing up, the sister with the enthusiasm, energy, laughter, and sharp thinking, was gone, replaced by a depressed, unenthusiastic, unhappy person who spoke of things in negative terms. After reading her chapter, you can plainly see that she now has boundless energy, enthusiasm, and a lust for life, all because she has been taking real hormones for ten years. I am so thrilled to have her back again.

One of my husband's dearest friends is also going through the same thing. He was one of the guys my husband used to hang out with in London in the sixties; they partied hard, played hard, and played around (I'm glad I wasn't in the picture at that time). They were two good-looking guys with the world at their feet. Now, though, the differences between them are startling. While Alan has, of course, become more mature as he has aged, with the friend you actually see an old man. Alan couldn't be any healthier or happier—he just glows. The difference between the two men is hormones: my husband is on bioidentical HRT, the testosterone patch and DHEA, and the friend is not. As you will read in chapter 23, Alan cannot say enough about the way he feels on hormones versus the way he felt before them. It has had such a positive effect on our marriage. Between the two of us, we have unbelievable energy and a zest for life.

There is so much confusion out there about this time of life and taking hormones. All I can say is, what have you got to lose? If you take real hormones under a doctor's supervision and find balance through blood tests, it's like getting a second chance at life. To go through the second half with the acquired wisdom and perspective, *and* balanced hormones, is a pretty wonderful experience. If you add to that mix a true change in your thinking about eating properly to keep your hormones balanced, exercising daily, and getting proper rest, you can change your second half of life to be the best it's ever been.

I am asked all the time what I do to look so healthy, and I always explain that I have found the fountain of youth in real hormones. Most people turn off immediately. Everyone has preconceived notions about hormones and aging. There have been so many con-flicting stories, and flawed incomplete studies, no wonder everyone is scared and confused. It is difficult to find the right doctor. But after reading this, you are better prepared to ask the right ques-tions. You never know where you will get your information. I found my doctor through my manicurist. I was complaining to her about my problems and she mentioned that she had heard of this doctor in Santa Barbara—one little mention that changed my life. This passage of life takes work, but hasn't everything you've strug-gled for in your life? Getting on track hormonally is worth the effort. The great thing about endocrinology is that you really have to go to the doctor's office only the first time. Since everything is assessed through blood tests, your relationship with your doctor can be maintained mostly by phone. This is a good thing, because after your hormones are balanced you will have so much energy, you will have trouble fitting another appointment into your busy schedule.

PART IV

THE
MALE
menopause

"Old" is when . . . getting a little
action means you don't have
to take any fiber today.

22

TESTOSTERONE AND MEN

So you think you are in this alone? Well, ladies, your men are going through male menopause, called andropause. It's real, and men truly suffer in silence. It is not a subject discussed in men's magazines. No man wants to talk about declining testosterone levels because it is so tied up in who they are. Without testosterone they aren't "manly."

It's unfortunate that people equate testosterone levels with the ability to have erections. Yes, testosterone levels do indeed affect the quality of erections, but that's the last thing to go; the real issue is loss of general vitality. I noticed this with my husband. His energy was gone—he was wilting like a tulip without water. He'd fall asleep midmorning, then again after lunch, and then again after dinner. I began to worry about him. We went to our internist in Los Angeles, who is a Western, Eastern, and holistically trained doctor. He has turned many people's health around, including mine, and I have great respect for him as a professional. He is of the new ilk of cutting-edge doctors who use Western medicine as a last resort. When an antibiotic is warranted, as with an infection, he is right there for you, but with a virus he prefers to use vitamins and supplements to build up the body's immune system so that you can fight the virus on your own. When I am overworked, he adds to or increases the supplements I take to give me more of a front-line defense.

We asked our doctor why Alan was running on empty. He

explained that because of our high-stress lifestyle, overwork, environmental pollution, damaged water, and damaged food supplies, including the damage that has been done to the soil that grows our food, it is necessary to supplement with herbs, vitamins, amino acids, and phytonutrients to make up for the poor-quality air, food, and water we now ingest.

Then we went to see Dr. Schwarzbein. After talking with Alan, she suspected that his hormonal production levels had dropped off. She had Alan take a blood test to review his hormone levels.

Well, lo and behold! My husband was almost out of testosterone. No wonder he couldn't stay awake. Testosterone is vitality, and without it one will not have the energy and zest to get through the day. Dr. Eugene Shippen says in his book *The Testosterone Syndrome* that loss of testosterone is at the core of male menopause (and a key element in female menopause as well). The two sexes have a different experience of midlife menopausal change. In women, there is an explosion of in-your-face symptoms, while in men very similar symptoms sneak in the back door. Most often, men's symptoms, such as loss of energy, ambition, and sexual drive, are written off as burnout or depression. Often, sexual virility is the last to go, so men don't think this "male menopause" applies to them—meanwhile they are drooping and sleeping the day away as my husband had been. Men feel as long as they can still "get it up" everything is okay, and put off going to a doctor. I look at this procrastination at getting help as precious time lost when they could be feeling their best. Because we women are barraged with uncomfortable symptoms, we go on the hunt for relief; because andropause happens to men over a ten- to twelve-year period, they usually chalk it up to natural aging.

Male menopause creeps up on them until finally they can't help but notice that their muscles are shrinking, their energy withering, their self-confidence crumbling, and their virility dropping off. The first sign that a man's hormones levels are dropping significantly is a subtle loss of strength and energy. There is also a depressive change in personality noticed by the wife and friends. There is often a loss of athletic ability, dynamic executive capabilities, self-confidence, eagerness, and aggressive energy, combined with a total unawareness of what they are undergoing. We all know men like this: those once high-spirited, energetic men who seem to have given up on life. A lethargy sets in. They are no longer interested in learning anything new, no longer want to join in the fun.

According to Dr. Shippen, "Men enter a gray zone, a time they neither understand nor wish to talk about." Male menopause is one of the most dynamic and significant events man ever experiences. His testosterone levels fall steadily decade by decade. Very few men have testosterone levels that stay at or near youthful heights right into old age. Dr. Shippen says, "I have never seen an older male in excellent mental and physical health whose testosterone levels were not well within the normal range. And the healthiest, most vital individuals are always in the high-normal ranges."

The changes that men are experiencing at this time are consistent with the hormonal depletion of aging. The optimal function of every cell in our bodies requires optimal hormonal input. Once we all had it, but as our hormone production declines, the result is suboptimal cellular activity. That is the beginning of trouble. It is subtle at first and usually thought of as natural aging, but long-term hormonal decline leads toward illness, fatigue, malaise, and further aging. Any doctor who looks for hormonal decline will find it in middle-aged women or men. Most of the major hormone systems drop significantly and steadily from year to year and decade to decade. It is one of the most important parts of the steady downward spiral into old age and debility. But now these lost hormones can be replaced in men's and women's bodies through bioidentical natural hormones, which results in rapid improvement in physical function.

Dr. Shippen writes, "The major controversy among physicians is whether gradual hormonal decline is a normal, healthy part of aging or is a pathologic, diseaselike state." According to Dr. Shippen, "This controversy sets up a false dichotomy. Hormonal decline is, of course, normal, but so is heart disease. They are also, and equally, disease states and will, in the end, prove fatal to any human being who allows either one to run its course unhindered."

There are many reasons why men, and women, too, should be wary of declining levels of testosterone. Testosterone is more than just a sex hormone—it is an anabolic steroid, which means that along with its unique chemical structure, it has the capacity to promote the formation of bone and muscle in the body. It travels to every part of the body. There are receptors for it from your brain to your toes. Testosterone is vitally involved in the making of protein, which in turn forms muscle. Testosterone is key in the formation of bone, and it improves oxygen uptake throughout the body, vitalizing all tissues. It helps control blood sugar, helps regulate cholesterol, helps maintain a powerful immune system. Testosterone appears to help in mental concentration and improves mood. It is also one of the key components in protecting your brain against Alzheimer's disease.

According to Dr. Shippen, "Without testosterone the muscle, nerve, and vascular systems that a man's sexual organs depend upon grow weak. Testosterone is also one of the most essential guardians of a healthy male heart. Testosterone is a muscle-building hormone, and the heart is the largest muscle in the body. In the human heart there are more cellular sites for receiving testosterone than in any other muscle of the body. Testosterone is also a stimulator of arterial dilation and increases production of nitric oxide, a natural form of nitroglycerin, the tablets heart patients take to open up the coronary arteries when angina pains arise. The pumping power of the heart decreases when testosterone declines, and angina pains begin when nitric oxide production declines. *When testosterone is administered in appropriate doses, most of the major risk factors for heart disease diminish.*" Dr. Shippen also says, "I find it puzzling that testosterone has not been given a prominent role in the treatment of heart disease. When testosterone decreases, cholesterol and triglycerides go up, coronary artery and major artery dilation diminish, blood pressure goes up, insulin levels rise, abdominal fat increases, estrogen levels go up, lipoprotein goes up, fibrinogen goes up, human growth hormones decrease, and energy and strength decrease, leading to a sedentary lifestyle and decreased physical activity. No other single factor in the male body is associated with more risk factors for heart disease than a lack of testosterone. Testosterone works protectively in men just as estrogen does in women."

Speaking of estrogen, men have to worry about their estrogen levels just as women have to monitor their testosterone levels. What? you ask. Here's the science, according to Dr. Shippen. The male body actually manufactures its own supply of the female hormone estrogen. It makes it out of its supply of testosterone. An enzyme called aromatase is widely present in the body and converts a certain portion of the male hormone into the female. The human body is expert at such processes, and actually the two hormones are chemically quite similar. This conversation is necessary for the healthy functioning of estrogen-sensitive tissues in a man's body. Estrogen is powerfully beneficial to the male brain. Too little estrogen will neuter a man just as effectively as too little testosterone. The areas of the male brain that control sexual function are plentifully supplied with the aromatase enzyme and thus have no difficulty converting testosterone to estrogen for its special purposes in those specific locations. Estrogen converted by aromatase can actually unlock or displace testosterone at its various cellular receptor sites. Too much estrogen will switch off activities. The body depends upon various on/off switches to regulate the force of its actions. Since testosterone is a powerful stimulant and energizer, estrogen may logically be a complementary "off" switch to turn down the male libido, as unbridled sexual energy can be totally disruptive to life. Whew! Enough with the science! But here's more . . .

Dr. Shippen says, "In older men, estrogens that rise out of their window of normal function become not a counterbalance, but a nearly permanent condition stuck almost always on 'off.' This is when effects on sexuality and a host of other male complaints become active." In many men, high estrogen levels cause a slow-down in testosterone levels. High estrogen levels can alter liver function, lead to zinc deficiency and obesity, and trigger alcohol abuse. High levels also increase aromatase activity. As a man grows older, he produces larger quantities of aromatase, the testosterone converter. Because of this, he converts higher levels of estrogen. Higher levels of estrogen can produce that "off" switch relative to sexuality. The liver eliminates chemicals, hormones, drugs, and metabolic wastes. Also among its duties is excreting excess estrogen from the body. Because too much estrogen in the male body has negative effects, it is important that the liver work at optimum. Zinc deficiency will adversely affect the male/female hormone ratio. Zinc is also important for normal pituitary function, without which the proper hormonal signals will not be sent to the testicles to stim-ulate the production of testosterone.

Both men and women require individualized quantities of both estrogen and testosterone to activate their sexuality and create all the other health benefits just mentioned. The good news is that now doctors in the know monitor this situation with HRT. As we age, hormonal changes are the single most important transforming factor for men and women. By replacing those hormones as you lose them, you can gain a reprieve from aging. They truly are the fountain of youth. This is what we have all been looking for: the magic potion, the secret elixir. And it's been right under our noses all along.

Having the means available to reinstate prime quality of life is an incredible breakthrough in today's medicine. I know that our mothers and our fathers, who pooh-pooh-ed this phase of their lives as nothing or hardly noticed, were just minimizing their expe-riences. The previous generation did not discuss their aches, pains, and complaints. It was partly pride, the "I will suffer in silence" syndrome of that era; also, there was nothing any doctor could do to give relief because so little was known about the endocrine system.

Now, not only are we beginning to understand a woman's need

for hormone replacement and the incredible benefits relative to quality of life and health, but also for the first time men can find relief for a problem that has been in the closet for so long. If life is not full of the usual zest you once enjoyed, perhaps testosterone may be the missing component. Every day I watch my husband, full of energy, taking two steps at a time on the stairs, leaping out of bed to start his day, on the phone, laughing, enjoying life, and running our businesses with a vigor I haven't seen in quite a few years. He is sold on the stuff. It has improved the quality of his life and therefore, in turn, mine. It all starts with a blood test to determine your levels; then read Alan's experiences in the next chapter to see how he is able to use this information to create a regimen with his doctor that works for him.

"Old" is when . . . "getting lucky" means
you find your car in the parking lot.

23

ALAN: A SIXTY-SEVEN-YEAR-OLD
MALE EXPERIENCE

My husband, Alan Hamel, is on bioidentical hormone replacement therapy, and I can vouch for the difference it has made in the quality of his life. It is like getting the "old Alan" back again. He has vitality, strength, and vigor. His mood is wonderful, he is mellow and in general all-around wonderful. He is so excited about the change in his personality and his sense of well-being that he would like to shout from the rooftops that he is on HRT. He has been on hormones for almost a year. Here are his feelings on the subject.

Before hormone replacement therapy, I was missing my usual energy and vitality. I was sleeping more than usual; and even after working out with weights regularly, I noticed my muscles were shrinking. I felt hollow. Also, my libido wasn't where I like it to be.

I have been on HRT for almost a year, and the results are amazing. My muscles are growing again, my vitality and energy are back. I don't feel exhausted by four o'clock in the afternoon, and I sleep more soundly. My mood is more upbeat and alert. My libido is once again my best friend [SS: "I'll vouch for that!"]. My brain is functioning and sharp again, and my general body functions have improved.

What I'd like to say to men is that they are looking for real trouble down the road by neglecting to look into the hormonal system relative to themselves. By not being proactive, they are turning their backs on a wonderful technology available for men. I don't look at HRT any differently from taking vitamins and supplements. Because medical technology is now keeping us alive much longer, nature needs a little assist. When I see my male friends not doing this, I feel sad for them as I watch them shrinking and becoming grumpy. I believe most men reject the concept of testosterone and HRT because they think it is an admission that they are not the "man" they used to be. They consider it a direct attack on their ability to perform sexually. I also believe that my HRT will help me to maintain a much better quality of life as I head down that lonesome road.

On a daily basis I slap on a patch that contains the prescribed correct amount of testosterone that my body needs. I also include a prescribed dosage, which at the moment is 20 mg once a day, of DHEA in capsule form along with my twice-daily ingestion of vitamins and supplements.

Because I am a firm believer in the mind/body connection, I am convinced that on this therapy my mind tells my body that it should be feeling great, and it always is.

"Old" is when . . . an "all-nighter"
means not getting up to pee.

24

DR. EUGENE SHIPPEN: ENDOCRINOLOGY AND ANDROPAUSE

Dr. Eugene Shippen, one of our country's leading endocrinologists, is the author of The Testosterone Syndrome. *Dr. Shippen is another of the cutting-edge doctors who are making a difference in the lives of thousands of patients who come to him as a last resort and leave after treatment with a renewed vigor for life. My husband devoured his information and was convinced that hormone replacement for men was also a valuable "edge" relative to longevity and vitality. Dr. Shippen is a great proponent of natural hormones and offers a fascinating viewpoint toward aging and how we can improve the quality of our lives.*

SS: Thank you for speaking with me, Dr. Shippen.

ES: Call me Gene.

SS: I loved your book, and I am particularly intrigued with your ideas of reversing the aging process.

ES: I'd rather say modifying it. "Reversing it" is a tough term, because part of the aging process is loss of cells. We lose so many brain cells, renal cells, so there is a decline that comes with the attrition of aging that we can't really stop. But we can certainly reverse the loss or decline of cellular dysfunction due to deficiency, and we can maintain optimal function. I look at it as though we are optimizing cellular integrity by maintaining signals to those cells, which in turn enables those cells to remain healthy. Hormones are the signals that tell those cells to burn insulin or do the million other things they do. So I look at it as a new way to maintain optimal cellular function through the aging process.

I don't particularly like the term *antiaging* because I think that people then assume we can live forever just by pumping in a bunch of hormones and turning our hormone levels back to what they were in our youth. That is too simplistic. My work is to optimize cellular function during the aging process before the aging changes have occurred. That way we create a much better environment for those cells so that they can regenerate and optimize the functional integrity of our body's systems.

SS: What is the biggest complaint you get from the men who walk into your office?

ES: Energy. And that's pervasive. It's an energy for life, energy for the things you used to like to do. It's energy in your brain to think clearly and be positively modified. It's energy for an upbeat mood and sense of joie de vivre. It's energy toward your mate. It's pervasive energy, not just fatigue. And it hits every part of the body because there are androgen receptors and estrogen receptors in every tissue. So your muscles are weaker, your joints are achier, your brain is not as sharp, your cardiovascular system is not as responsive, you're more breathless at tasks that didn't used to make you breathless.

SS: But I imagine that most men are not in tune with their lack of vitality; it's too vulnerable. So how do you pull this information out of them?

ES: I have a checklist, which basically looks at energy in every system of the body. For instance, mental, moods, musculoskeletal system, energy toward sex and sexuality, the prostate. A lot of the BPH (benign prostatic hypertrophy) symptoms that we get are due to a loss of energy of the prostate muscles that open and close the doors and allow flow to be maximized. A lot of the BPH symptoms don't correlate at all with the size of the prostate. They correlate with the testosterone. Once we make that link, men don't have to get up to urinate three times a night. There is a misconception among urologists that BHP is really due to enlargement of the prostate. Half of the men don't have an enlarged prostate, and the missing link is testosterone.

SS: So as men lose their hormones, testosterone in this case, they lose their muscle tone not only outwardly, but internally as well?

ES: Correct. Bladder function, prostate function, sexual function, and tone in the muscles of the pelvis are all related to declining testosterone levels and atrophy. They literally lose the athleticism of those muscles.

SS: I would think the biggest complaint that would get men to come to your office would be loss of erections.

ES: That's not the most common. But if you ask them, they'll say, "I'm doing fine." Then I say, "Well, how are you doing compared to when you were thirty-five?" I don't talk about when they were twenty-five. Those were crazy years. But think back to thirty-five, what was your frequency? If they were once- or twice-a-week guys, now they are once or twice a month. They say it's still working all right, so they don't necessarily see it as a problem. They are just more tired, or they are busier, or their mate is not as receptive, or one hundred other things. But when a man's hormones are in balance, meaning our libido is also in balance, we are always looking for windows of opportunity. Libido's a subtle thing and it's vulnerable, so frequently they won't complain of that.

SS: What are the other complaints?

ES: Things are happening that didn't. They will complain that "I'm failing when I didn't use to." So libido and sexual function are highly variable, something that you can't rely on as primary indicators. But pervasive energy changes. If somebody comes in not feeling up to par, you start to explore every part of the energies of life and you will find that low testosterone explains declines in all the energies.

SS: Do you find that men and women don't realize how bad they are feeling until they experience hormonal balance and it makes them feel better?

ES: Yes, because unless you know it's broken, you sort of accept the changes of aging as, "Okay, I'm over fifty, I shouldn't be running up and down the mountains in the same way. I can accept that." But when you fix them, and they start running up and down the steps and so on, and they get their zest for life back, and their energy systems are working again, it's like turning on all the healthy switches that you are familiar with.

SS: I see it in some of my friends—it's about their vitality. I see them slowing down measurably. . . . My husband gave one of his friends your book and he was offended. He said, "What's the matter? I don't have any problems." Is getting help difficult for men because it's all wrapped up in their maleness?

ES: You have no idea how truly bad it is. It's all wrapped up in our cultural expectations; the way in which aging men are portrayed is the way in which doctors have been telling their patients what to expect. I have patients I have put on testosterone, they feel better, they're doing better, and then they see their doctor back home, who tells them only about the dangers. So they stop taking it. And then they feel bad again, but now they are frightened, that to feel better now, they are going to have to pay some kind of price down the road.

SS: Is that true?

ES: Nothing could be further from the truth. It's the healthiest thing they could do. All you are doing is restoring back to normal what is no longer being produced.

SS: It must be terribly frustrating for you.

ES: It is. Men either reject the idea that this is really what they need, or they find another doctor who gives them the fear of prostate cancer, or the unknown. We don't have long-term double-blind studies to show that it is healthy, but my answer to that is if we used that same filter for everything, we might as well stop practicing medicine. No drugs have those kinds of documented benefits for over ten years—where double-blind randomized control studies show that they are safe and efficacious for treatment. Even with statins, the drugs that lower cholesterol, we don't have ten-, twenty-year studies.

SS: You mean like Lipitor and Pravachol?

ES: Right. These drugs may lower your testosterone at high doses. So from my standpoint, these people are running a grave risk of actually decreasing their health in the long term. In the short term they may have fewer events for unknown reasons, but there's no improvement in long-term mortality with these drugs.

SS: As a female I take bioidentical hormones. Is that what you use for men?

ES: Absolutely. I would never use a substitute. All the substituted forms are the ones where we've had bad effects. There's a good reason for that. When you substitute a hormone, it is not metabolized into other hormones the same way. I give testosterone in its natural form. Our body can then convert it into estrogen. As we age and get chubbier, our bodies may produce too much estrogen, and estrogen in men is one of the most important by-products of testosterone. A substitute form of testosterone, like methyltestosterone, cannot be converted like natural testosterone. Only bioidentical hormones will be handled by the body in a natural way, allowing it to balance these secondary hormones in a healthy pattern.

SS: So many women are automatically put on synthetic pharmaceutical hormones at their first complaint. If they are antisynthetic, then the next remedy is black cohosh or eating a lot of yams. Initially this happened to me, and I was in such of state of zeroed-out hormones that I wanted to tell my doctor where to shove those yams, because yams and black cohosh were not giving me any relief.

ES: I say black cohosh is great if you're a geranium, but if you are truly deficient it won't help if you are human. It doesn't provide you with the estrogen benefits on bone and cardiovascular. There's no proof that it does any of this. In fact, there is growing evidence that black cohosh and other herbs are so weak, they're only covering up some of the subtle symptoms to make women more comfortable.

SS: Then there's soy. Women are downing those soybeans like jelly beans. They're eating tofu (soy is the new buzzword in health food stores), and they are shoving so much soy into their systems, but it makes you think, doesn't soy promote estrogen production?

ES: It has some activating effects.

SS: If so, isn't it a little dangerous to activate estrogen, because you are creating an imbalance?

ES: Well, yes, that's true. Let's go back to the estrogen receptors. There are two different kinds of estrogen receptors, maybe more. It's well known that there are estrogen alpha and beta receptors. One receptor activates the other. In other words, phytoestrogens can be used for one effect, but the other effect is having some benefits and some side effects. We don't know whether the phytoestrogens activate or block. In small doses soy may activate the receptors in one way and in large doses may end up blocking them. The way I approach it is to consume small amounts of foods to provide the phytoestrogens that have always been in the food chain.

SS: What other foods have estrogenic capacity?

ES: How about clover? You can look at all of the different plants and they all have estrogen to some degree. To overload one type, to kind of force-feed the body to take a very high concentration of soy estrogen, is going down uncharted waters, and it's not a substitute for the natural bioidentical estrogens that are metabolized and balanced in the body.

I try to take a balanced approach. The Japanese get somewhere around 50 mg of phytoestrogens daily from the food they ingest, and I wouldn't take any more than that. But I will tell you this: If I could change something in my book, it would be soy for men. When I had men taking soy, I found it to be helpful.

When we are young, our liver can clear estrogen very efficiently. As we age, lean body mass goes down, fat cell mass goes up, and the circulating testosterone gets converted in greater amounts into estrogen in our fat cells because of enzyme activity in fat cells. If you look at individuals, you'll find that chubby guys who have central obesity (thick through the midsection) are high in estrogen. You'll find the greater the obesity, the greater the number of fat cells, the greater the conversion of testosterone. Where there is a greater conversion of testosterone to estrogen (and men hate to hear this), estrogen proves to be a more powerful hormone to them than testosterone. Estrogen is highly regulated in a man's body. So the estrogen says to the pituitary, "Hey, we've got a lot of estrogen here, so let's turn down the production of testosterone."

SS: But does this extra estrogen provide protection for the man's heart?

ES: On the one hand, it might provide protection for the heart, but as estrogen gets too high, the blood has an increased tendency to clot. One of the studies on heart disease shows that men who have heart attacks have higher estrogen levels and lower testosterone levels. The ratio gets reversed, and the thinking is that maybe increased estrogen increases the likelihood of forming a thrombosis in the coronary arteries.

SS: Is balance the key?

ES: Balance is the key. There are guys who want to get rid of every bit of estrogen. They want to be pure male. I tell them the ying yang is alive and well. Without estrogen there is no libido. There was a study that showed that men who did not produce estrogen had osteoporosis, heart disease, and low libido, yet they had testosterone levels that were two to three times normal.

SS: Why do they do movies called *Grumpy Old Men*?

ES: The studies on mood are so highly variable that it's hard to draw broad conclusions, but I will tell you this: If somebody has never been depressed, and at middle age starts to become depressed, measure his testosterone levels, because the depression won't go away until you correct his testosterone.

The number of men I treat with depression almost always get better with testosterone replacement. Many of them had been on antidepressants and did not get better.

SS: So a man might go to a psychiatrist for his depression when, in fact, all he needed was to restore his testosterone level?

ES: In a lot of cases, yes. The problem is that once they get on antidepressants they're married to them forever. They feel they can't live without their antidepressants, but antidepressants further depress their testosterone and they don't really get better. So now they are constantly in treatment. But when you ask how they were when they were thirty-five, they could slay a dragon.

SS: Do you feel that testosterone is a means of staving off disease?

ES: Absolutely. The linkage between disease and testosterone has been totally overlooked. It is well documented in literature. Almost every disease drives testosterone down. Testosterone is anti-inflammatory, it's rebuilding, it's anabolic, it's good for insulin. It's good for maintaining all the things that get suppressed in most common diseases—inflammatory disorders, arthritis, asthma, heart disease. The information on heart disease relative to testosterone is absolutely astounding, and it's totally ignored. You can give a shot of testosterone to a man who has coronary artery disease and he'll last a minute longer on a treadmill without changes in the cardiogram. It has an immediate vasodilating effect on the coronary.

SS: Does it have any effect on lungs, or people with emphysema?

ES: Absolutely, yes. And here's another thing: Colitis gets better when testosterone levels are checked and testosterone is administered. Colitis is treated with steroids; as soon as you start taking steroids for colitis (corticosteroids, prednisone), testosterone just drops dramatically. Then a man starts losing muscle mass, he gets weaker and weaker. He loses his insulin sensitivity, he starts to gain weight. Steroids knock you down physically, and testosterone will actually reverse and protect you.

SS: What about DHEA?

ES: I don't give DHEA to anyone who doesn't need it. One of the problems is that they never do double-blind long-term studies looking at this kind of medicine that fixes two, three, or four things at once. So if you just do a study on testosterone and that person is low on DHEA and low in growth hormone, and his thyroid is out of balance, he is not going to have the same benefit from testosterone as another person. You have to look at every one of those parameters and fix them. When you do you'll find that the person responds to testosterone with renewed zest for life and will get his energy back.

Diet is crucial and essential for good health. All the HRT in the world will not do the good it wants to do if you are eating badly. Dietary patterns make a huge difference in our likelihood of getting cancer. There's a supplement that helps the metabolism even more, and it's called omega-3 fatty acids.

SS: Yes, I take that two times a day.

ES: The Japanese get high amounts of DIM (diiodomethane) in their vegetables and a high amount of fish oil in their fish. Yet it's amazing: if they move to our country, they get the same breast cancer or prostate cancer, because they begin to eat our diet, which doesn't have enough omega-3s, and we do not eat the same amount of cruciferous vegetables.

There are other things . . . minerals. Selenium is very important. There are three well-documented things that I look at for modifying the risk of cancer. One is indole-3-carbinol, or I3C, which comes from cruciferous vegetables, and the omega fatty acids help with that. The other is vitamin D, which has been shown to have an effect on estrogen metabolism in a different way. It turns estradiol back into estrone, which is the weak estrogen. When that system is working, the body has the ability to regulate estrogen according to its needs, instead of being overdriven toward the more powerful estrogen, estradiol.

SS: I didn't realize vitamin D had that effect.

ES: Yes, it also has the ability to induce cells that are becoming cancerous to self-destruct, plus it has some anti-inflammatory effect. Vitamin D in adequate doses protects bone from osteoporosis. So vitamin D is helpful in lots of wonderful ways—its anticancer effects, its benefit as an anti-inflammatory, its influence on estrogen metabolism, and its ability to induce cancer cells to self-destruct.

The other important supplement is selenium. Selenium is now being studied in a test with fifty thousand men for its ability to prevent prostate cancer. But selenium has already been established as a useful supplement against breast cancer and colon cancer. In animal testing, selenium reduced tumor replication and had a variety of therapeutic effects on different kinds of tumors. So I put all my patients on selenium. Women should be taking selenium because of the risk of colon cancer as much as breast cancer.

SS: What about antioxidants?

ES: Despite what the cardiologists say about antioxidants (which is that they are not good for anything), I do believe antioxidants are important, along with folic acid and the natural antioxidants.

SS: There's a lot of controversy about HGH [human growth hormone].

ES: I'm very careful with HGH. I test for IgF1, growth factor. If it's low, I test for output. I always do a challenge test. I never give HGH just as an antiaging supplement just because theoretically it's useful. But endocrinology brings in people who have been everywhere else and haven't found relief.

SS: I believe in today's world your endocrinologist is your most important doctor.

ES: Some of them are like frightened sheep unless they're on the cutting edge. Most endocrinologists are very conservative, and they're waiting for the world to move them. I like to live on the cutting edge. I love science.

SS: Me too. I never knew I would be fascinated by physiology.

ES: Well, it's the creative application of science. When people say, "What do you practice, complementary or alternative medicine?" I say, "No, I practice innovative medicine." The only new patients I take are those who are interested in innovative therapy.

For instance, from the standpoint of my research, if you have breast cancer, and you go on hormone replacement, you are no more likely to have a recurrence than a woman who doesn't take it.

SS: Where were you when I was being chastised by the press for taking hormones with my cancer? *People* magazine did a cover story asking, "Is she risking her life?"

ES: If you do get a recurrence or a new tumor, it will most likely be estrogen-receptor positive, which is far less aggressive. So you'll have a better chance of surviving it. Additionally, if you are on bioidentical HRT, your colon cancer risk will drop by 30 to 35 percent, and that's a bigger killer for women. Colon cancer is more likely to kill you. It's the hidden cancer, whereas breast cancer is out front. Breast cancer is 90 percent curable if caught early, and colon is only 45 percent curable; it depends upon the stage, but you are much more likely to die from it. There is a 30 percent reduction of colon cancer risk if you are on bioidentical HRT.

SS: Well, that's great news. Please tell the media, so they can stop scaring women to death about HRT. The reported studies are terribly flawed because they are done with synthetic, pharmaceutical hormones.

Now what do you tell men about bioidentical HRT?

ES: I tell men there's no connection between maintaining normal testosterone levels and prostate cancer, and this has been well supported in literature. The difference between getting cancer in men is diet and lifestyle, as evidenced by Japanese men having less prostate cancer than we do. So they are doing something that doesn't make colon cancer grow and gobble us up. Some of the things that are healthy for us, relative to the study of men and prostate cancer, will in the future be far more beneficial than doing PSA tests and biopsies on men.

SS: What's the future? Where are we going?

ES: In the future, I hope that scientists realize that the complexity of the human organism doesn't always lend itself to long-term double-blind randomized studies. It's time doctors started treating people as individuals. In doing so, there will be massive reductions in all the major degenerative diseases as we normalize hormones, normalize nutrients, and key in on lifestyle, diet, and environmental factors.

I think our capability for living out our normal genetic life span will be greatly enhanced through bioidentical hormone replacement, by keeping all of our functions reasonably intact: our brain, our motor system, our ability to get up and do the things that keep us self-sustaining late into life.

SS: So you're talking quality of life.

ES: Yes, maintaining that general quality of life and maintaining all the functions that we hold dear, sex included. I have some ninety-year-olds who are enjoying that side of life. It's just our perception that sex is no longer important when you are old. We can't envision our grandparents making love, but it's a perception. Balanced hormones give you vitality, and sexual vitality is part of it . . . that is, if science doesn't bog us down with fear over the lack of these long-term studies.

SS: Thank you, this was enlightening. And keep doing the good work. Ever since my husband got on bioidentical HRT, his vitality has returned. I've got my old (young) guy back.

beating
THE
clock

"Old" is when . . . going braless pulls all
the wrinkles out of your face.

———

25
PHYSICAL AGING

Okay, this is the crummy part. Who likes to wake up each day and find that another part of their body has dropped? You already know I think the best way to fight physical aging is getting your hormones balanced. Finding balance for me has been like finding the fountain of youth. It has allowed me to forget all those symptoms that were beginning to plague me before I started balancing my hormones. But no doubt about it, the body shows its wear and tear around this age. I have become philosophical about it. I have decided to change my take on it. I focus on how great I am looking for my age. I never expected to look this youthful at age fifty-six. Really, when I think about the women of my mother's era, we have great advantages today that were not available to them. One of the first big advantages is that we now know how to take better care of ourselves. We are the first generation of women who have really embraced exercise. We understand nutrition better than ever before; yet, even armed with this knowledge, many still choose to eat foods laden with chemicals and preservatives. Nothing will age you faster than ingesting chemicals. Simply put, aging results when our bodies break down more cells than they build up, and chemicals will certainly break down your cells.

My friend Dr. Schwarzbein says that as a society we are on a frightening accelerated metabolic aging path. If you have read any of my Somersize books, you know what I'm talking about. Bad eating habits, stress, caffeine, alcohol abuse, and inactivity can lead to extended periods of high insulin levels, which prematurely ages our bodies on a cellular level. This aging process leads to disease. Additionally, when the hormone insulin is present in increased levels, it can disrupt every other hormone system in the body, which can lead not only to excessive body fat, but also to degenerative diseases of aging such as different types of cancer, cholesterol abnormalities, coronary artery disease, high blood pressure, osteoporosis, stroke, and type 2 diabetes. Most people do not realize that hormone imbalances always lead to disease. Furthermore, women who are already going through menopause are at extreme risk of disease.

As women age, we naturally become more insulin resistant, which explains why it gets harder to stay slim as we get older. Adopting a high-carbohydrate diet exacerbates the problem because all those carbohydrates increase insulin resistance. The elevated amount of insulin in the blood increases testosterone levels, which further blunts the production of estrogen and progesterone, the female sex hormones. Compound the problem with a low-fat diet and you have even less hormone production, because we must consume real dietary fat to create hormones. Besides the uncomfortable side effects of hot flashes, cramping, and mood swings, an imbalance of these sex hormones means we cannot produce healthy cells! It is at this critical stage that women become vulnerable to disease.

This is the connection among nutrition, health, and aging. Everything we put into our mouths, good or bad, has a direct effect on our health and, thus, our ability to stay youthful. We all know eating junk food is bad for us, yet I don't think we consider the consequences of the bad food choices we make. Years of poor eating habits cumulatively add up to damaged cells and our bodies' inability to produce new, healthy cells. When we eat poorly, we age faster, not only externally, but internally as well. This accelerated metabolic aging process leaves us vulnerable to disease at an earlier age. Eating right isn't just about weight loss, it's about total health that determines how well we age. Most important, we can control our bodies' ability to combat the diseases of aging when we understand the connection between the intake of real and healthy foods. It doesn't matter what you have achieved or how much you have earned or what titles you have held. If you don't have your health, you have nothing! (Oh, God, did I just say that? I hear my grandfather's voice in my ear.)

In my Somersize books, I constantly drive home the importance of eating real foods to lose weight; but we need to stay away from processed foods and trans fats for another important health reason. Processed foods introduce free radicals into our systems. It is important to understand the consequences of free radicals.

Free radicals are molecules that carry an extra electron. Since electrons need to be paired off, these free radicals roam through our systems like little home wreckers, trying to steal electrons from healthy cells. This process damages our systems on the cellular level. Antioxidants, such as vitamin E, vitamin A, and vitamin C, help to neutralize free radicals. But when we replace real food (which includes natural vitamins) with processed food, we are not supplying our bodies with the natural antioxidants we need to fight the free radicals; instead, we are introducing more free radicals into our systems! The damage that results over time accelerates the metabolic aging process and leads to insulin resistance, then disease and possible early death. Ironically, two of the most powerful antioxidants, vitamin A and vitamin E, are found in foods that contain real fats. Unfortunately, the fat most people consume is unhealthy fat, like trans fats that come in bags of potato chips and corn chips, or processed foods with ingredients that no one can pronounce.

Processed foods and trans fats aren't the only things compromising our health. Consider that the average American consumes forty-three gallons of sugary soft drinks every year! We are literally killing ourselves with sugar and chemicals that break down our bodies on the cellular level. The sugar and caffeine in one cola wreak havoc on the body by spiking insulin levels. Think about that every time you consider having a can of soda. The average can of soda contains one-quarter cup of sugar. Imagine eating one-quarter cup of sugar in its dry form—you would gag. Yet most of us drink several cans of these sodas every day without even thinking of the amount of sugar we are ingesting and the effect it's having on our insulin levels.

Imagine the insulin in your body looking unsuccessfully for places to store the abundance of glucose from all the sugar we ingest, whether it's in the form of cakes and cookies or high-starch vegetables or white-flour pastas or white breads. Then visualize how the sugar gets converted into fat because your cells just cannot accept any more sugar. Visualize the free radicals sweeping through your system and damaging your cells.

With diet drinks you don't have the sugar to contend with, but you have the additional free radicals from the artificial sweeteners. The most recent studies on the effects of aspartame (NutraSweet, Equal) are frightening. Lab studies have proven irreversible brain damage in laboratory animals. In fact, one can of soda can raise the levels of toxins in the brain of an infant higher than levels that caused brain damage in immature animals.

I apologize for laying all this physiology on you, but I think it is important to understand the effects of food on our bodies, especially at a time in our lives when we are no longer producing a full complement of hormones, which as I have said leaves us vulnerable to disease. Part of looking good and feeling good is internal health. I also want you to understand the importance of healthy cell reproduction.

This is why, when I was diagnosed with breast cancer, I was so adamant about continuing hormone replacement therapy and did not want to take chemotherapy if there was any way I could avoid it. I knew that chemo would destroy my healthy cells along with the unhealthy ones, and I felt it was a greater risk for me. I know already that as I get older, some of my cells will die off; and there is nothing I can do about that. But I also know that if I am not giving my body the proper combination of nutritious foods, my cells will die off at a more rapid rate. When I feed my body properly, my cells thrive; and I feel empowered knowing I can stave off disease and aging for as long as possible. Healthy cells will keep you young, slim, and looking great.

We are going to age physically, no matter what we do; but we do have control over how we age and how well we age. Look around at the seniors you know. Which ones are in the best health? It's those who have always exercised and eaten properly. I'm not talking fanatics, just those who kept a check on themselves. There is no free lunch. You get out of life what you put into it. That's just the way it goes. The reason some people look better than others is that they work at it. That's the reason celebrities look so extraordinary. They are constantly thinking about their appearance because it is their livelihood. They are in the business of making pictures, whether it's on television, in magazines, or in the movies. Celebrities know that they have to stay fit and healthy if they are to make a living. Eating real foods instead of processed foods, avoiding chemicals, exercising daily, drinking lots of water, getting plenty of rest, watching the consumption of alcohol, and avoiding smoking all add up to looking great. Granted, it's easier to pull into Jack in the Box and order a burger, fries, and a milkshake; but it will show on your hips, in your skin tone, and in your overall general health.

It takes more work and discipline to look good as you age, but you are the beneficiary. When you look around you, it is easy to see those who have given up. It happens to both men and women. First comes the weight gain that accompanies middle age. Weight will keep piling on if no thought is given to controlling it. I know many once thin women who let it get out of hand or did not understand the effects of insulin resistance during this passage. After the weight has taken hold come the various diseases associated with aging.

Most people simply expect that disease is part of aging and have no understanding of the effects of elevated insulin levels (eating too much sugar). Aging and disease do not go hand in hand. Bad lifestyle habits are the culprits in aging. If we could truly grasp that we are in control of our health, that it is not necessary to spend our last years in hospitals or with oxygen tanks or with limbs that can no longer hold us up, we would make the necessary changes immediately. Being ill is a terrible way to spend the second half of your life, and it isn't necessary. You have the power to change the course of your life. It's a choice, but it starts now. If you wait much longer, you will have gone past the point of no return. As they say, this isn't a dress rehearsal, this is the show! We can have life and vigor right up to the end, but it's up to each one of us to choose. And that's what it is—a choice. Have your cake now or choose to beat the odds.

Here is what it takes—*commitment!* It requires that you say to yourself, "Today I am going to change my habits." Then you have to mean it. Once you have truly made a commitment, it gets easier. When the alarm goes off in the morning, don't lie there all cozy and warm. Designate how many days a week you have decided to exercise and then do it. Try doing something that you enjoy. It is not necessary to join a gym and commit all your time and money to exercising. Just find a way to get moving. Physical activity releases stored sugar from your cells. As soon as that stored sugar is released, your body starts burning off its fat reserves. That's when you will start losing weight and your beautiful body will start revealing itself.

You don't have to be a fanatic. I exercise every other day (every day when I am in training for a tour), and I do this at home. I spend twenty minutes doing cardio. I like to walk up and down my outdoor steps ten times (about twenty steps). That really gets my heart rate up.

Then I use free weights for another twenty minutes, and then I do mat exercises—squats, leg lifts, pushups—and waist exercises. I do use several of my own exercise products (ThighMaster, Bodyrow, UltraTrack), but you can get the same results by stretching and doing situps (it just takes a little more effort). Machines force you to be in the right positions, which can make exercise easier and more focused; an improperly performed exercise has little to no benefits other than cardio. And with the timers that are often on machines, you get motivated.

Take the stairs instead of elevators, walk to the store rather than drive, play tag with your kids, swim, jog: all of these are easy and enjoyable ways to get fresh air and exercise. Notice that the older people who are fit and in good health are always the ones who have eaten good food in moderation and were conscious of doing some kind of exercise every day. Exercise feels good, it puts pure oxygen into your bloodstream, it promotes good health and fitness, and it's good for your bones.

Rethink how you eat, too. For breakfast, instead of having a bagel or a muffin (cake in a muffin cup), have a fruit smoothie and fresh eggs and sausages or a healthy and great-tasting breakfast cereal with nonfat milk. Drink decaffeinated coffee; caffeine lowers your serotonin levels, which then makes you crave comfort foods, usually carbohydrates or something sugary. The body accepts carbohydrates, particularly refined white flours, as sugar; so drinking caffeine eventually will make you fat. Besides, caffeine blocks estrogen production, which eventually leads to insulin resistance, which also makes you fat (and bitchy, I might add) and will lead to disease . . . all for a cup of coffee? Try Starbucks' Guatemalan decaf. It's delicious and strong, and you'll suffer no adverse effects.

It's these simple first changes that will set you on a path of healing and good health. Watch and see how quickly you are pleased with what you see in the mirror. As I said, the choice is yours.

Perks of aging: Your joints are more
accurate meteorologists than the
National Weather Service.

—

26

BONES

As we age, we hear over and over to take calcium to protect our bones, and for the most part we are pretty good about remembering to take those capsules every day. But have you ever considered how diet affects your bones? What would we be without our skeletons? A pile of jelly! The food we consume from childhood throughout our lives will directly affect our bone structure. At menopausal age, we women start to worry about our bones. Our doctors tell us to have a bone density test. Most of us have already experienced bone loss. We accept this; in fact, we expect this to be the case. But hear this: Bone loss is not a condition that has to accompany middle to old age. Osteoporosis is insidious because you can't see or feel it happening. Most people who have the disease don't know it. And then a bone breaks or fractures.

Each year 430,000 Americans wind up in the hospital because of fractures related to osteoporosis. Hip fractures, which represent about 300,000 of that total, are devastating. One victim in five dies within a year, and half are never able to live independently again. Most of us know someone who has suffered a hip fracture, but you may be surprised to learn that complications of the injury kill even more women every year than breast cancer. Preventing osteoporosis is really a life-and-death matter, like preventing cancer and heart disease.

Hip fractures are just the most obvious part of the problem. Millions of women suffer distressing symptoms that they don't connect to fragile bones. A woman may not realize that her chronic back pain comes from crush fractures in her spine. Fragile vertebrae may have crumbled under the ordinary stresses of everyday life. Osteoporosis can make a woman look old before her time, but she may have no idea that her slumped posture and protruding tummy are caused by fractures in her spine. As a woman you have one-in-three odds of suffering from osteoporosis in your lifetime. You can beat those odds. Medical experts now consider osteoporosis a preventable disease. Osteoporosis is treatable thanks to new findings about nutrition and exercise, as well as new medications and hormone replacement therapy.

Even women in their twenties and thirties can get osteoporosis. Fortunately, this doesn't happen often, since most early victims of the disease have significant risk factors such as prolonged use of steroid medications or lengthy periods of eating disorders. Ironically, many of these women are dancers or athletes who look healthy and fit. The bones we have later in life reflect what we did as kids, teens, and young adults. So in a very real sense, osteoporosis is a disease that starts in childhood. Consider this when you hear of a teenager who is struggling with anorexia. The immediate and long-term effects are devastating. This is why it is so important that our children eat healthy right from the start. What they put into their mouths now will affect not only whether they are overweight or obese later in life, but also how healthy and strong their bones are. If a woman is menopausal or premenopausal, extra calcium can help build strong bones. But simply upping calcium consumption has never been shown to increase bone density or prevent fractures in older women. Add vitamin D to that calcium and the effects are dramatic: bone density increases significantly, and fractures are reduced by 50 percent. That's because vitamin D is needed to absorb calcium and turn it into bone, and many postmenopausal women don't get enough.

Going on HRT using bioidentical hormones can also help build bone strength. Estrogen replacement has been shown to help prevent osteoporosis, and you get this benefit from taking estriol as part of HRT.

Here's something you probably didn't realize: Men also are prone to osteoporosis. An estimated two million men have this disease. In fact, a man is far more likely to suffer an osteoporosis-related fracture during his lifetime than he is to get prostate cancer; yet men, and even their doctors, are largely unaware of this problem. Hormonal stimulation is just as important for men's bones as it is for women's. Low testosterone levels are responsible for about half the cases of osteoporosis in men. Usually, low testosterone is a consequence of aging, but certain medical conditions can lead to more rapid loss. Signs of low testosterone in men include the following: reduced libido or impotence, decreased facial and body hair (for a woman it is increased facial and body hair), and enlarged breasts (although many men have low testosterone levels without any symptoms at all). A blood test can measure testosterone levels. If you are low in testosterone, ask your doctor about a bone density test.

Men with a light frame and low body weight and also men with eating disorders are particularly at risk for osteoporosis. Competitive athletes in sports with weight classifications especially suffer from the problem. Anyone who has been a yo-yo dieter or had anorexia or bulimia is at a higher risk for osteoporosis. Other risk factors for men and women are inactivity, a diet low in calcium and vitamin D, high alcohol consumption, and smoking (current or past).

Here's what you can do to restore your body and your bones to good health:

1. **NUTRITION:** *Eat real foods, and enough of them. Remember, food is fuel, which you need for energy, and real foods promote healthy cell reproduction. In addition, real foods promote strong healthy bones.*

2. **PHYSICAL ACTIVITY:** *Be active. Weight training in particular promotes bone growth. Here's how. When you do weight training, the muscles tug against the bone, promoting and stimulating bone growth. The outward physical benefits are*

also apparent. Nothing is more beautiful than toned, defined,
cut muscles. Your clothes will look better on you, but the
inward effects are the most exciting benefit. You will be
building bone or, in the case of bone loss, restoring bone.

3. **SUPPLEMENTS:** *Take calcium, vitamin D, and Fosamax (if*
necessary, depending upon your bone loss). This, of course,
should be discussed with your doctor.

4. **HRT:** *Continue to take estriol as part of hormone replacement*
therapy under your doctor's supervision.

Perks of aging: People no longer view you as a hypochondriac.

———

27
SUPPLEMENTS

Here is the next big thing regarding antiaging: supplements. What a difference it makes to supplement your diet with all the nutrients, herbs, vitamins, phytonutrients, and amino acids that our body needs for survival but in general most of us are missing; they are absolutely life changing. I used to wander into health food stores and gaze at all the vitamins stacked in their neat little rows and wonder what they were all for. At times I would make a feeble attempt to take a "one a day" vitamin, but aside from that I was pretty unaware as to their benefits. I think it is vitally important to find yourself a cutting-edge doctor who is interested in the antiaging approach to life and health.

I never knew anything about this approach to health until after my mother passed away. I experienced terrible grief upon losing her, but my work schedule left me no time to grieve. In fact, the day after I buried my mother, I was on the Home Shopping Network for nineteen hours over the weekend, and my work continued at that pace for several months. Before long, I began to have health problems. I felt as if I were wilting. I couldn't stay awake. I would fall asleep in the car on the way to meetings or work, struggle through whatever it was that I was required to do, and then sleep all the way home. I would walk into the house (it was multileveled, with many stairs), and whereas I used to bound and leap, two stairs at a time, now I had to sit and rest before I could contemplate heading up to the bedroom. If I awakened to go to the bathroom in the middle of the night, I would have to sit and rest halfway to the toilet (and my bedroom was not so big). I felt as if I were slowly running out of gas. I had no energy, I was overly tired for my age, and I couldn't understand because I was on bioidentical HRT and eating properly.

What I hadn't factored in was stress. Stress causes most of our problems. For sure stress blunts hormone production, so even if you are still making a full complement of hormones, acute stress is going to affect your levels. How could I have thought that the loss of my mother, who is the reason I am sane today, was something I could "get over in time"? This stress, along with a lack of nutrients because our food supply is damaged, as well as contaminated water and air, plus my body's inability to operate properly because I was still so upset from my mother's death, coupled with being run-down from overwork . . . and *duh!* No wonder my body was shutting down! I was ignorant of the fact that grief is a process and must be dealt with just like any emotional problem—and will not go away until it has been. I wrongly figured that my sadness would go away "in time."

Soon it was becoming intolerable, and I felt my abilities to work were being compromised. I went to see my internist, who, as I mentioned before, is a Western, Eastern, and holistically trained doctor. He did some tests and confirmed to me what I already inherently knew, that my adrenal and cortisol levels were completely burned out. Besides that, I had developed something called "leaky gut," a precursor to Crohn's disease. This meant that I had developed little leaks in my upper intestine from stress and that the toxins from my intestines were leaking into my bloodstream, which was literally causing me to break down and wilt. I had never felt so fatigued—just walking to the doctor's office exhausted me. We talked for a long while, and after I explained about my mother and my workload and my inability to take any time to come to terms with my grief, he figured that I had gotten this ill because I had not dealt with the pain of losing her. He lectured me about balance, and I felt embarrassed because I know these things; but, of course, the messenger does not always live the message.

Every test he took came up low or depleted. It was this doctor who started me on a regimen of vitamins and herbs. I began with a pharmaceutical-grade multivitamin, calcium and magnesium, folic acid, coenzyme Q_{10} (which carries oxygen to all the glands, including the adrenals), glucosamine (because I complained about joint pain), vitamin C (1,000 mg), Eskimo-3 fish oil and omega-3 fatty acids for the heart, Flora Source to fight yeast, and Adrenal 180 (because my adrenals were blown out).

Throughout the year, he continually changed the amounts depending upon my workload and stress level. When called for, sometimes he added extras, sometimes he took away. It all depended upon my strength and energy. I must say, since taking all these supplements I rarely get sick anymore, and I feel an inner strength I never had before. Even though I am in glorious health today, I continue a regimen of supplements and vitamins as a first guard against illness and as a means of building up my body's strength.

In addition, Dr. Schwarzbein has put me on more supplements and amino acids: Sam-e, St.-John's-wort, and L-tryptophan for depression, irritability, PMS, and carbohydrate cravings; evening primrose oil and L-glutamine for additional help with carbohydrate cravings; carnitine to decrease carbohydrate cravings and mobilize fat; L-tyrosine, which relieves stress on the adrenal glands (tyrosine converts to adrenaline and aids in the functioning of the adrenals); L-taurine as a diuretic, along with vitamin B_6 for salt and water retention; and lecithin, glycine, and phosphatidylserine for irritability and anxiety.

My friend and master herbalist, Paul Schulick, who produces high-quality herbs and supplements for his company, New Chapter of Vermont, sends me the following: Smoke Shield for smoke exposure, air pollution, and exhaust fumes; Rhodiola, which improves mental, immune, adrenal, and cardiovascular performance; green and white tea capsules for longevity, heart, and immune system function (these contain health-promoting antioxidants); Host Defense, which enhances human natural killer cell activity up to 300 percent; Zyflamend, which reduces inflammation; Holy Basil to deliver nutrients to the mind; and Turmeric Force (turmeric is one of the world's most important healing herbs).

On my own, through a lot of reading, research over the Internet, and talking with several cutting-edge doctors, including my own internist, I found Iscador, to fight the cancer that has already invaded my body. Currently I am NED, no evidence of disease, but I was looking for the most palatable way to fight against the return of this cancer. Iscador is an anthroposophical medicine made from plant extracts, developed by the famed homeopath Dr. Rudolph Steiner in the early 1920s in Europe. It has been used at the Steiner clinics in Europe in place of chemotherapy, and they have had the same results, with no side effects. Iscador is not an FDA-approved drug in this country, so I am not suggesting that you go the same route. I will not know for another two years if Iscador has done all that the manufacturer, Weleda, said it would. I will keep you posted. I inject this extract, made from mistletoe that is grown on special types of trees (it's unlikely that the one you hang above your doorway at Christmas is what they are talking about), every other day, and I will continue to do so for the next two years, while I am still in the danger zone. I so believe in its healing effects that I am considering taking Iscador for the rest of my life. The manufacturer claims that it will build up the immune system, protecting it from invaders such as cancers, which of course is very exciting to me.

I know this seems like a lot of supplements to take, and maybe I am going overboard, but it does show that working with doctors who are "in the know" allows you to get as involved in supplements as you care to be. You should create your own program, but I thought you'd like to see my regimen as a means of comparison. As I said, this particular passage takes more work if we want to have a great quality of life. With the environment as damaged as it is, we have to be proactive about our health. We are not getting the proper nutrients from our food anymore because of the damage that has been done to our soil, air, and water. We ingest chemicals most of the time without even knowing it. Our food supply is contaminated with chemicals and toxins. What are we to do? We can sit idly by and talk ourselves into thinking we are impervious to such things, but I have already had my first scare, which I now consider to be one of the many blessings of cancer. I can't fight the damage done thus far to the environment, so I am taking the first line of defense, by making my body "war ready." At least if I get polluted with chemicals and free radicals by unintentionally ingesting foods that have been contaminated (and face it, when you have to eat in as many restaurants as I do, I am bound to be getting some polluted food without knowing it), at least I can fight back by building up my immune system through supplements, vitamins, herbs, and Iscador. It's all I know how to do.

Do I like taking this many pills in a day—no. But I do care about living a long, healthy life, and I don't know any other way to do it. I am not alone in this. All my doctors concur, and so many doctors who are up on things are turning to supplements as a first line of defense. The new cutting-edge doctors understand that our lives today are not as they were when older doctors were in medical school. We have reached contamination levels of unprecedented proportions in the last several decades.

Recently, I hemorrhaged my vocal cords by overusing them in rehearsal. I went to my throat doctor in a panic, because I would be doing previews for my new Broadway show in four days. He shook his head and said that normally it takes ten to fourteen days for vocal cords to heal, but if I rested my voice completely until then (not a single word), perhaps I had a chance. I returned to him four days later, quite anxious, as you might expect. He looked at my vocal cords on X-ray and said, "This is a miracle. I have never seen such a fast recovery; it must be all the supplements you take." I was able to do the previews in perfect voice. It's little things like this that give me the incentive to take all these ingestibles each day.

If you feel that supplements would benefit your health, start asking around. Get the names of the most advanced or cutting-edge doctors in your town or city. Recent med school graduates have accepted integrated medicine as a normal part of health care. You might find out from one of them where to go for help. Having a Western doctor is a must—in the end, we need to rely on drugs in an emergency—but check around to find out if there is a doctor in your city who also heals through supplements and herbs. A doctor trained in Eastern and holistic medicine along with Western is best of all. Often that doctor has an office on the same floor with an acupuncturist or a massage therapist. This approach to medicine is deliberately integrated and collaborative. You may be asked to turn off your cell phone, to keep the waiting room calm and serene. As a result, this may turn out to be the one time in the day when you can get that quiet. What better way to walk into your doctor's office? Your calm demeanor allows him or her to get to work right away. You've had time to think about why you're there. You can develop a meaningful relationship with your doctor this way.

Perks of aging:
You can eat dinner at four P.M.

28

RITA: A SEVENTY-YEAR-OLD EXPERIENCE

Rita is another inspiring woman, full of life and energy and good feelings. It's truly remarkable to talk with a woman of seventy years who is so progressive, because she comes from an era (as my mother did) that accepted doctors' advice as dogma. To go against the grain and partake in something as cutting-edge as natural bioidentical hormone replacement is not only forward thinking but courageous. After talking with Rita, I became more convinced than ever that natural hormone replacement is the way to go. This is a woman who is enjoying her life, and she is as sharp as a tack. Read for yourself. . . .

SS: Good morning, Rita, and thank you for speaking with me. I know you are a patient of Dr. Schwarzbein's, and I was very interested in knowing how you feel, having been on natural hormones for such a long time.

R: I feel great! I entered menopause at age fifty-five. At first I was on synthetic hormones for a few years, and I felt awful. I was depressed, tired, I had constant headaches, my breasts were always swollen and tender, and I was puffy all over because of the water retention, so I just stopped taking the hormones because I thought, I can't feel any worse.

SS: Then what happened?

R: I started to feel as if I were living in someone else's body. I couldn't relate to myself anymore. You know what I mean? My body just didn't behave or react as it had for all the years before menopause. I was pretty discouraged.

Then I heard about this young endocrinologist in my area who was prescribing natural hormones, and everyone who was taking them was talking about how great they were feeling. So I thought, It can't get any worse than this, and I decided to make an appointment.

SS: How long did it take after you started on natural hormones before you began to feel any difference?

R: Almost immediately. I felt more energetic, and my depression was gone. Life was beautiful again.

SS: Tell me about your typical day.

R: Well, I wake up early, around four o'clock, but I wake up so happy I just like to lie there and think good thoughts. Then usually around six A.M., I get up and get ready for work. I teach Spanish at the university. I have worked all my life, since I was seventeen years old. My students all think I am young, and I like it that way. They guess at my age, and usually they say that I am fifty or sixty years old. But I think it's because I have a youthful energy. It's been this way ever since I have been on natural hormones. They make me feel more energetic. I take care of my two grandchildren quite often, and what's great is that I have the energy to be with them. I've always had a lot of energy, I have always been very active; but when I was on synthetic hormones, I just lost my zest for life.

SS: So what is your teaching schedule like?

R: I schedule classes from eight A.M. until noon every day. Two days a week I give two classes in the afternoon from four until seven.

I try to exercise as often as I can. I walk every day and on the weekends. I have a stationary bike that I use quite often, and I move constantly.

On weekends, my husband and I do a lot of things together. We enjoy each other's company. We go to restaurants, or the beach, or we take a lot of drives.

SS: What about sex, if you don't mind my asking?

R: We are still enjoying sex from time to time. It's not the way it once was, but I think ever since I have been on natural hormones, my feelings have come back. When I was on the other hormones, there was a lot of vaginal dryness. That does not make it fun. But now that is gone and sex feels good again. I think my husband should be on natural hormones. He is in his seventies also.

SS: Do you still have a period?

R: Yes, I do. I had a lot of bleeding last year because I had fibroid tumors. So I stopped taking the natural hormones, and then I started to feel awful again. The biggest thing I notice is that my brain stops functioning well when I am not on the natural hormones. So I went back on them, had the fibroids taken care of, and now things seem back to normal.

SS: But doesn't it bother you to have a period at this age? Isn't it just a hassle?

R: No, it really doesn't bother me. It's worth the trade-off. I feel so much better when my hormones are balanced. It's the difference between really living and just existing. So what! I have a period. I also have a brain, and that is more exciting to me than worrying about having a period each month. Besides, when Dr. Schwarzbein explained to me that having a period is the most natural way to go through this passage, it made sense. We are mimicking my normal physiology. That seems right.

SS: Do you take vitamins and supplements?

R: Yes, I do. I think they are very important. My body is working well. I am not stiff and I don't feel old, so I assume that all these things I am doing are making me feel that way.

SS: Are your friends taking natural hormones, or synthetic hormones, or nothing at all?

R: Some of them take nothing, some of them are on synthetic, and I can see the difference between them and me. None of my friends work, they can't think, they forget everything, and they are slow. Whenever I am around my friends, I am thankful that I have a brain that is together. Good brain function is the best part of all of this. I am seventy years old, and I am enjoying my life. I don't want it to be over. I think taking natural hormones gives women a second chance. My life is so good, I can't really remember what it was like before. I am so involved in my present circumstances. I went from being depressed, crying, and miserable to having energy, vitality, and clear thinking, and my zest for life and my work is back.

SS: How long will you continue to take these hormones?

R: Forever. These hormones have changed my life. If my doctor told me that I had to stop them, I'd say, No, no, no! And again, the greatest advantage of taking these hormones and supplements is my clear, sharp, functioning brain. I remember things. My brain is working great, and that is a huge thing.

SS: So you are enjoying this second half?

R: Enjoying it? It's better than the first half was. My relationship with my husband is better, my entire situation is better. When I was young, I had too many problems. Even my husband and I had reached a point where we had just gotten used to each other, but now . . . Wow! We're having a ball!

SS: How great. Is there anything else you would like to say to women?

R: Don't be afraid. Find a good cutting-edge doctor who really knows what he's doing. If you don't, you are the one who will suffer.

SS: Thanks so much. You are wonderful and an inspiration.

Perks of aging:
Kidnappers are not very interested in you.

29

DR. MICHAEL GALITZER: NATURAL HORMONES AND ANTIAGING

I have probably sent more than one hundred people to Dr. Galitzer, and without exception everyone loves him. A girlfriend who was on a series at the same time I was starring in Three's Company *has had chronic medical problems and she finally found relief through Dr. Galitzer. He found that everything troubling her medically was hormonally driven. Dr. Galitzer believes in natural bioidentical hormone replacement; he believes in approaching health holistically, using the best of Eastern, Western, and holistic medicine. Dr. Galitzer's enthusiasm is catching. He takes the mystery out of aging; through instruction, and working together as patient and doctor, the second half of life becomes the enjoyable passage it was designed to be. You will enjoy what he has to say.*

SS: Antiaging medicine is very exciting. Would you explain exactly what it is?

MG: Antiaging is about maximizing energy. I would equate lack of energy with accelerated aging and maximizing energy with slowing down the aging process. If I had to assess someone quickly, more than blood tests, I would tell them optimize your nutrition and optimize your emotional state. By doing those things, you will ultimately optimize your energy and feel younger.

SS: I believe natural bioidentical hormones are the fountain of youth we've all been looking for. What importance do you place on hormones relative to aging?

MG: When patients come to me and complain about lethargy, that they just don't have the same energy or the same sex drive, I try to explain it to them from a hormonal point of view, because I think that puts everything into perspective. The key hormones to start to work on are the adrenals; they sit on top of the kidneys and are most affected by stress.

SS: Stress blunts hormone production, so you would first check the adrenals and then the sex hormones?

MG: Right. In the body the adrenals represent survival, whereas the sex hormones—progesterone, estrogen, and testosterone—basically represent reproduction. To the body, survival is always more important than reproduction. So the body will do whatever it takes to maximize adrenal hormone output and survival. With that in mind, the body will convert the sex hormones into adrenal hormones to maintain survival at any cost, which is why when you are stressed and tired, your sex drive goes down. So you really can't go straight to the progesterone, testosterone, and estrogen before you look at the adrenals. You've got to maximize the adrenal.

SS: How do you do that?

MG: There are lots of ways these days that you can evaluate adrenals—with a blood test, with saliva, or with something called heart rate variability.

SS: What is heart rate variability?

MG: Essentially, the more variable your heart, the more each beat is slightly different in length from the preceding beat, the greater the variability, the healthier the autonomic nervous system. The autonomic is the subconscious nervous system, the autopilot of the body that controls things we don't have to think of, like blood pressure, pulse, and breathing. When you do a good history, you find out that people with weak adrenals get tired around four o'clock in the afternoon. They sometimes get a little dizzy when they stand up, and they also might crave sweets. Most people have weak adrenals, and in some people it is more important than in others.

SS: That's interesting. I was experiencing dizziness for a period of time when I got out of bed in the morning. My doctor had me go to an ear, nose, and throat specialist, but at the same time he said my adrenals were blown out and gave me supplements to rectify the matter. I thought the ENT doctor made the dizziness go away, but now I am realizing that it must have been the adrenal supplements.

MG: Right, there is something new called metabolic typing. There are four basic metabolic types: the slow oxidizer, the fast oxidizer, the parasympathetic dominant, and the sympathetic dominant. What this basically says is that there is one system that helps maximize energy in each person. So if you are a parasympathetic dominant, your adrenals are the key system. If you are a sympathetic dominant, your thyroid is your key system. If you are a slow oxidizer, it is your pancreas.

SS: I think you will have to explain that one.

MG: Okay, say you are a parasympathetic dominant, which means your adrenals are key for maximizing energy and processing energy in your body. If you have weak adrenals you are in big trouble, because basically that is your key system and your key system is out.

This happens in pregnancy. For example, when a woman is pregnant and she is stressed in, say, the sixth month, she will start converting her own progesterone (of which she is making lots during pregnancy) to the adrenal hormones. In month seven, the baby's adrenals kick in, and the woman starts stealing from the baby's adrenals; so the baby's adrenals start revving up to supply the excess adrenal hormones that she needs. Then at birth they cut the cord, so the lady loses her fix and suddenly goes into postpartum depression. The child may then become hyperactive and get colic and all those other things. It is part of the process.

SS: Tell me about cortisol.

MG: Cortisol and DHEA are the two hormones made by the adrenals. Initially when you are stressed, cortisol levels go up, and if you are the kind of person who takes stress home, you take that stress back to the family and have a hard time sleeping. The reason you have a hard time sleeping is that cortisol levels are very high at midnight, and that turns off melatonin and also turns off growth hormones. Growth hormone is secreted in the first two hours of sleep, which really allows for the physiological regeneration in the first half of your sleep. If your cortisol levels are high at midnight, you are not going to sleep very well, and you will wake up not feeling well. So it's important to get the adrenals under control because so much is affected by them.

SS: Yet because of a lack of understanding, most people in this situation would be prescribed sleeping pills when in fact, they might have an endocrinological problem having to do with the hormone cortisol.

MG: Yes, but more important, we have to look at the adrenals first. The adrenal cortex, which is the outer part of the gland, makes cortisol and DHEA. If a person has already gone into first-degree, second-degree, or third-degree stress (massive stress being fourth-degree), when the next stressor comes on, there is no third-degree cortisol or DHEA to be released because the adrenals are shot. So what does the body do? It goes to the adrenaline. The adrenaline is not where you want to be.

The body does not have enzymes to break down the adrenaline. Adrenaline is your last-ditch effort. This can cause people to get very anxious and feel palpitations. Adrenaline also has a real affinity for the joints, so people will have weakness or stiffness in their joints, all triggered by blown-out adrenals.

SS: Women are confused about menopause and they don't know where to go. There are conflicting reports on HRT, but all the studies are done on synthetic hormones. How are you taking care of menopausal women?

MG: First of all, very tenderly. But it is science, and I get to work finding out all that I can about her history. When a menopausal woman comes to me, I take it that her progesterone and estrogen are not very high, so I do a complete hormone check, but I would also like to know the status of her adrenals. The other thing I do is a BTA—blood, urine, and saliva. We look for pH and redux; most people have acidic tissue, which is reflected in an alkaline blood pH. So the higher the pH is over 7.35, the more acidic the tissues are. I usually see 7.55, 7.58, 7.60, which generally represents an enormously acidic body.

What occurs is that the liver is out to lunch. The liver is the major cleansing organ of the body. The danger with an acidic body is osteoporosis. When the tissues become acidic and the body has to neutralize acidity, it steals calcium and magnesium from the bone, which is the greatest reservoir to neutralize cellular acidity. So if you have an acidic body with a liver that is not working as efficiently as possible and estrogen starts to accumulate in the body, you have a woman who is set up for estrogen dominance. Normally people are acidic because of a very sluggish liver, or a poorly functioning lymph system, or it could be they are not drinking enough water. Many of the foods we eat are full of estrogen, pesticides, and insecticides. And let's not forget those mercury-silver dental fillings.

SS: What would mercury fillings have to do with a woman in menopause?

MG: The mercury behaves as estrogen in the body, so you get a kind of setup where you have a sluggish liver and an estrogen level that's too high relative to progesterone. Mercury is one of the biggest problems. The older the fillings the more they leak, and they leak to a certain threshold point over years, and that is when symptoms occur. The mercury the dentist puts in your teeth must be put away in a special container that says "Poison" on it. That should tell you something. Root canals are in a different category and one of the few areas in medicine where dead tissue is retained within the body. You can cut out a person's gallbladder or appendix, but with a root canal, the nerve root is dead but there are so many tiny canals in one single nerve root that it is almost impossible to keep all the canals completely free from infection. So the thinking is that some of these canals are still infected and the infection is able to seep through the bloodstream to other areas. Plus, each tooth is connected to an organ, if you are using the meridian system. So frequently a root canal tooth—say, the upper molar—would connect to the stomach meridian, which connects to the thyroid and the breast. Are you still following me?

SS: Yes, and I am fascinated.

MG: Progesterone usually sinks first in a woman. It can start at age thirty-five. So if you have a person in her forties with not enough progesterone, who is affected by the toxic environment and has mercury fillings, plus too much estrogen, and if the woman is overweight at this point (fat cells make estrogen), what happens is estrogen dominance, which I think is the major player in both breast cancer and prostate cancer.

SS: But innovative integrated antiaging is more than a medical workup, isn't it? New medicine treats body, mind, and spirit.

MG: You are right. So when a woman comes to me, I do testing, but I also ask many questions such as, Do you drink coffee, alcohol, Coke, tea? Do you eat pork, bacon, ham, breakfast sausage? Do you smoke cigarettes? What kinds of medication are you on? Do you ingest sweeteners like Sweet'N Low or Equal? Do you eat lots of fruits, do you eat lots of vegetables? Do you eat a lot of sugar, and do you crave salt? Do you have PMS, do you exercise, do you drink enough water, do you take supplements? Do you have any root canals, and do you have silver fillings?

Then I go a little deeper: Do you meditate? How is your relationship with your significant other? Do you like your work? What is your purpose in life? Why are you on planet Earth? Do you feel connected to God or a higher power? What is your support system like with family and friends? Are you having enough fun in your life? What we put into our bodies, what we think, how we live our lives, the relationships we have, all have a major effect on our health. When someone says to me, "I am not happy in my life," I try to find out what makes her or him happy. What turns you on, what excites you? If I had to look at it, I would say the three major areas are to be happy, to be of service, and to experience who you really are. Certain people may have a different order of what is most important, but the big question is, where does one find joy? I think most people don't really realize that the main purpose in their life is to be happy.

SS: If this person has not been able to find joy in her life, do you recommend counseling?

MG: Yes, we have so many wonderful tools at hand today. Therapy can turn people's lives around. The people who are not happy are really not clear about their purpose. I think you have to look at whom you are spending your time with. Most people spend time with their significant other or with the people at work. If both of those are not working, I think it's going to be pretty hard for a person who isn't that conscious to get out. Antiaging medicine is full-service to mind, body, and spirit. I don't think you can slow down the aging process if you are not balanced emotionally. When these questions are answered, I am better equipped to treat this person because I have all the information. Joy in one's life is nature's best healing antidote. Today we can work together as doctor and patient for maximum results. We are living longer than ever before, and the second half, as you call it, can be the best if we appreciate and value the incredible machine we have been given to house our mind and spirit. But it all works together and cannot be discounted as irrelevant.

SS: What are your feelings about natural bioidentical hormones?

MG: I think natural bioidentical hormones are essential. I think they are essential in creating longevity and slowing the aging process. Obviously reducing toxins and reducing tissue acidity are also important, but the endocrine or hormonal system is the one that most connects with how we feel. The hormonal system is what most correlates to the emotional person; it is not the liver or the kidneys. Basically, the hormonal system is most affected by our emotional state, and it is clear that the hormonal system responds to our outlook on the world.

SS: Wonderful information. Thank you so much.

MG: My pleasure.

Perks of aging:
Things you buy now won't wear out.

30

EVE: AN EIGHTY-YEAR-OLD EXPERIENCE

As much as I enjoy the quality of life I am experiencing on natural bioidentical hormones, I have wondered (a lot) what it is going to be like to have my period when I am in my eighties, and is it worth it? Well, here is a woman in her eighties, still having her period and a full, rich, vital life. I was very anxious to talk with her and found her to be the most inspiring role model. She verified for me that it's a small price to pay for the zest and vitality that she is enjoying. I loved talking with her and learned a lot about the important things in life.

I am eighty years old and feel great, but it wasn't always this way. I was married most of my adult life and have two beautiful children. They give me such joy. I am a recovering alcoholic, sober for thirty-nine years, and at age sixty-five I fractured my back. As I lay in bed for weeks, I felt scared to death that I would never be able to work again. I didn't want to end up bed-ridden, like my daddy. At the time, I had already been through menopause and had not taken hormones because my Tulsa doctor at that time told me I didn't need them. There was no incidence of heart problems or stroke in my family history, just TB and pneumonia; so my doctor said that hormones were not important for me. After I fractured my back, my doctor told me it was because I had lost so much bone, so maybe now I should take Premarin, a synthetic hormone.

I had heard negative things about synthetic hormones from my friends, so I did not want to take them; but after a year in physical therapy, I realized I had to do something. My osteoporosis got worse and I panicked. I decided that I was going to really look into alternative medicines. I felt as if I were starting to fall apart; looking back, I now realize I was. I gave up coloring my hair and wearing nail polish. I tried to avoid chemicals wherever I could, thinking that these things might be contributing to my poor health.

Everyone in Santa Barbara was talking about this endocrinologist Dr. Schwarzbein; some thought she was fantastic, and some thought her theories were crazy, but I heard she was doing natural hormones and I went to see her. I was impressed from the start. Here was this tall, vivacious, good-looking woman with shiny, clear eyes. All I could think of was that I wanted some of what she had. She put me on natural hormones, and I began to notice a difference right away. I felt the urge to be active again. I believe that energy begets energy, so I started to walk every day. I also got into meditation. In my meditation I have rituals: Father, I greet you; I am a radiant, healthy woman. And then I would visualize myself as that woman. I would visualize myself as tall, erect, with good posture. I think good posture is so important; if you've ever fractured your back, you'll understand how desirable it is to have good posture.

My internist was distressed that I was taking these hormones at my age, but I believed in my new doctor and trusted her. To look the way she does, she must be doing something right. And on top of that, I was feeling so much better than I had in years. I began to exercise. I could feel that my bones were strengthening, and my energy was so different. My thinking was back in focus. I felt sharp and in tune.

My friends thought I was crazy because I was having my period again, but I didn't care. I figured it comes with the territory. I was growing bone again, and I was feeling so great. Some months I would bleed more heavily and I would call Dr. S. and say, "Is this for real?" Then we would do another blood panel to find that my hormones needed some adjusting. At my age, things are changing so fast that we need to pay careful attention. I don't use tampons. I don't know, I just can't get used to the idea. My daughters keep trying to encourage me to use them, but I am more comfortable with Kotex.

Today, fifteen years later, I feel great. I have so much energy and joy. I wake up early every day, but I lie in bed until around seven A.M. The first thing I do is make my bed. Once you reach your seventies and eighties, it's easy to fall in love with your bed. So I get up right away and I dance while I am making my bed. I usually listen to Roy Orbison or the Beatles. I do facial exercises for my neck and chin, and I make a promise to my body that I will take good care of it today. Happiness is what this is all about. Since I started with natural hormones, I feel happy most of the time.

I go to exercise classes three days a week. Some of my girlfriends go to these classes for social reasons, but not me. I have a purpose. I am taking care of myself. Exercise is so important; you know, if you don't use it, you will lose it. It all has to do with energy.

After I make my bed and dance, I have coffee (real coffee)—it's my only cup of the day; then while I am making my breakfast, I watch David Letterman. I tape him every night and watch him in the morning because he makes me laugh. For breakfast I usually have yogurt, half of a bran muffin, one-quarter of a Fuji apple, and shredded wheat with milk. Then I either go out or I sit at my computer and go to my Web page. No one reads the stuff I write, but I don't care, I enjoy getting my thoughts down. Once a week I go to line dancing. I love it. There are a lot of nice men there, and we have a lot of fun.

My girlfriends my same age don't have the kind of energy I have. When I walk, I bend and stretch. It feels good. I believe we have a healer within us, and I also believe that exercise is vital. I promised my body that I was going to take good care of it, and that's what I am doing. I lie down for a nap at two o'clock, but I never go to sleep. I just rest. Then I get up and watch Dr. Phil. I really like him. There's something vicarious in watching him. He forces you to really look at the truth about yourself.

I admire Dr. Schwarzbein because she is a front-runner. She has courage and is willing to step out and dare to be different. She gets a lot of criticism, because she is cutting-edge. She has made this her specialty.

I don't have a sex life. I carried a torch for my husband for a long time. But I do still have sexual feelings. I just learned my testosterone is low, so we're going to adjust that. Not so that I can have a stronger libido, but for hormonal balance. It's a good thing my testosterone is low; otherwise, I might be out there walking the streets [laughing]. Regarding men, I do love to hug them and kiss them. I don't care if they are bald or if they are good-looking, I just want them to have good, clear eyes.

I drink about six glasses of water a day, plus one more at night when I take my Metamucil. Yes, as you get older you do have that problem, but I find dancing and exercise really help. For lunch I always have protein and some carbohydrates. I usually have raw vegetables also. Dinner is salmon, a little pasta, and a salad. Right before I go to bed, I have hard rye crackers and maybe some herbed cream cheese and part of an apple.

I am not stiff, I do not have aches and pains, and if aches do come, I refuse to entertain them. If I miss a day of walking, I feel things stiffen up a little. I enjoy laughing. I think we have to laugh at ourselves. I do three Kegel exercises three times a day. It's funny. I have a cat and he is my pal. I talk to him as though he's a person. I never liked cats before. I grew up on a farm and was one of twenty-three kids, so we never had room for any pets. My cat keeps me calm. He's part of my ritual. I never was a *Leave It to Beaver* kind of mom, but I find myself saying, "Hi, I'm home," to him when I come in the door, and it is a nice feeling.

I feel so much of my well-being is because of these hormones. I stopped taking them at one point because they are expensive and when you are a senior every cent counts (it's about $65 a month plus), but after three months I couldn't stand it anymore and I went to the doctor to put me back on hormones.

I plan to continue taking these hormones. It's the sense of well-being—I have to attribute it to that. My body is different from those of other people my age. My thinking is sharp, I read a lot, I'm happy, and I'm satisfied. I have a lot of zest and energy. I look forward to each day. I would say to other women, Try it for six months. What have you got to lose? Don't knock it till you've tried it. I think the mind-set is very important. I feel that I am a well person. Another part of my ritual is that I read anything about being well or staying well. I have a happy attitude, I feel fortunate, I have beautiful children, and I feel each day that God blesses me.

PART VI

living an
AUTHENTIC
LIFE

Approximately 85 percent of all American
adults are walking around with
burnt-out adrenals, and they deal with it
with Prozac and coffee!

———

31

WHAT YOU DIDN'T GET

The other day I was observing someone I know very well and thinking about the difficult time she was having in her adulthood. It is clear from my vantage point that at the bottom of her trouble is what she "didn't get" in her childhood. I think that is what runs all of us. From outward appearances she had an idyllic childhood, yet upon close examination, was it really? She lived in a beautiful home with a swimming pool, a nanny, and all the creature comforts. But these things will never make up for the unhappiness that pervaded her childhood home. Her parents had a loveless relationship, and when that relationship exploded and they succumbed to divorce, she was left without a proper explanation from either parent and spent the rest of her formative years living with a very angry mother who took shots at her father at every opportunity (a classic situation, by the way). Her mother's anger became her own, and they lived in angry harmony for the rest of the years spent together.

This is a typical scenario in today's modern world. Divorce is the inheritance of this new generation. In my younger years, I was the first person I knew of in my little hometown who was divorced. It was quite a scandal; so much so that I finally had to leave town and move away to escape the whispers and the gossip. Today, divorce is a normal, albeit unhappy, occurrence, something that is more accepted, and the child of divorce does not stand out as he or she once did. Nonetheless, it is not any easier to cope with.

When childhood anger goes unchecked, the result is a chaotic adulthood. As I said in an earlier chapter, the pain you experience as a child does not grow up and mature, even though you do. When the anger or pain of your childhood is not dealt with, it remains locked in your soul and becomes a driving force inside you. One of the most important things you can do for yourself as an adult is confront the pain of your childhood. I grew up with the notion that "the past is the past; let it go." Ah, that it could be so easy! You can move on, but the pain will not. It stays and smolders and is the basis behind your short fuse, or those unexplained moments when you weep for no reason, or the bitterness you feel in general toward life, or the jealousy you can't seem to keep in check. You don't want to be this way, but these feelings are the motivating force behind everything you do. It's embarrassing and difficult to admit even to yourself, because it manifests from something that happened so long ago.

Until you deal with them, these feelings will sit, lying in wait, to ooze out of you at the strangest moments. A good way to discover the driving force behind your unexplained moods is to pay attention to the times when you "lose it." What is it that made you so angry with your husband this morning? (Of course, if your hormones are not balanced, that could explain everything.) I know my buttons are pushed whenever I feel that control over my life is being taken away from me, even a little bit. If my husband makes a plan without consulting me, and it hits me at the perfect hormonal moment of the month, I can get irrationally mad. Why? Obviously I still have more emotional work to do relative to the complete control my alcoholic father had over my life.

So control issues still push my buttons. What are your issues? What makes you emotional? What is the line in the song that your heart responds to? What is the part of the movie when the tears come rolling down your face? Pay attention to these things. These feelings are you talking to yourself. Feelings are how we teach ourselves. Feelings are ourselves trying to let go and release, yet rarely do we pay attention. We just chalk it up to external circumstances—the movie was a tearjerker, or the song was very emotional. But our messages come to us in mysterious ways, through the lyric of a song, a scene in a movie, or a sentence in a book.

Next time it happens, ask yourself, What feeling does that trigger? Take a few moments to think about it. This is not a trivial exercise. These are our opportunities for clarity. We are run by our past until we have dealt with every part of it. You don't need to have been an abused child, as I was; everyone has people and events from the past that are life defining, and often these events are precisely the parts of our lives that have undermined us and made us feel inadequate or unworthy.

What didn't you get in your childhood? Ask yourself this question, and be honest with yourself. After all, this *is* for you! You are old enough to handle it now. Did you not get enough attention? Did you feel you were taking up space in your childhood home? Did you have siblings who taunted you? Did your parents divorce without explanation, and somehow you thought that if only you had been a better child, you could have saved the marriage? Do you feel responsible for some traumatic event that happened in your past? Did someone in your family become very ill and you thought somehow you were responsible? Was one (or both) of your parents abusive, or alcoholic, or a drug abuser? Did you have parents who didn't seem to notice your existence? Do you feel that your parents didn't want you or need you in their lives? Have your relationships not worked out? Were you abandoned? Did your parents not accept you as you are? Do you not have satisfactory relationships with your grown children? There are hundreds of reasons for our unhappiness or our inability to put our finger on happiness. What it eventually comes down to in almost every situation, after peeling away layer after layer (and this can take years or a lifetime), is that you didn't get the love you wanted or thought you should get.

So much of why I am a happy person today has to do with the emotional work I have done in my life to undo the damage of my childhood. I never got the love I wanted or thought I should get from my father. He loved his bottle of booze more than any of us—addiction does that. It took me years to find forgiveness for my father. I spent three years in intense therapy, trying to understand why I had such low self-esteem, why I didn't feel good about myself, and why I was insecure in the presence of just about everyone. Because of this intense therapy, I finally got to the bottom of this force that drove me and had shaped my personality. It was difficult and agitating work. At times I wanted to run from it because it brought back all those buried feelings with full intensity; but I stayed with it, and it is clear to me today that this is the single most important thing I have ever done for myself. Without having done the "work," my life never could have taken the turn that it did. I never would have had the self-esteem to pursue my career, never would have felt worthy of my wonderful husband, never would have learned to love my father for being one of my most important teachers. Through his disease, I was forced to either make a life for myself in spite of the disadvantages of being raised by him and his alcoholism or become a victim of it. I chose not to be a victim, and then I went to work. What a great choice. Because of this choice, I was able to turn his disease around to my advantage. Had I not chosen this path, life as I now know it would not exist. In fact, my self-esteem was so damaged that I question if I would even be alive today.

If this rings any kind of bell with you, think about those things in your life that are in your way. Think about what you didn't get in your life. Generally, we are embarrassed to hearken back so long ago, to times and events that today seem like nothing. For many of us, there are obstacles in our lives (some big, some small) that can trigger years of buried feelings that have been in our way. The object of this glorious age, these fabulous forties, fifties, sixties, seventies, and eighties, is to get the most out of this second half. Finally we have time for ourselves to figure out who we are and what we want. These are big questions and won't be answered easily. It has taken half a lifetime to develop into the person you have become, and if, at this age, you are not happy with that person, it's going to take some time to change into someone else. But it is so worth it! The next fifty years await you, and how glorious they can be if you let go of the negative times and events that have been running your life. There is such freedom in looking the past in the eye and choosing to fix those parts of yourself that have been damaged as a result of a past you haven't wanted to remember. The result is an authentic life. When you are living an authentic life, the only person you are accountable to is yourself; the only goal is to do the right thing for yourself. It is hard work, and will require focus and attention until your very last day, but what graceful work it is.

Perks of aging: Your supply of brain cells is finally down to a manageable size.

32
CONCLUSIONS

By now, I hope I have convinced you not to be afraid of this passage and not to dread it. I stated at the beginning of this book that this is the best I have ever felt and that I have never been happier, menopause and all.

No doubt about it, this passage requires management and handling, but the rewards are worth it. Bioidentical hormones give you an edge over aging never before experienced, if for no other reason than to retain optimal brain function. I don't know about you, but I never want to lose my abilities to think and dream. A great functioning brain is a true gift as we head toward old age. But as you know from reading this book, replacing lost hormones with natural bioidentical ones gives you an edge in almost every area of your life. Hormones are life!

Thank you for going on this journey with me. This is the book I was looking for when I first entered menopause, but it did not exist. Everything I read pointed out the negatives. I dreaded menopause, and in my first year of this passage the quality of my life was drastically altered. I went on this search for myself, and after going through hundreds of books and studies and talking with many doctors, I was finally able to figure it out. There is no perfect doctor out there; the field is too new. There is too little understanding among doctors. That is why you have to be proactive and get this information for yourselves. We are the pioneers in managing menopause, and our daughters will have an easier time

of it because of us. It makes sense, because we are the first generation to live long enough to see menopause all the way through. If
you do nothing, you will be the loser. I am enjoying every day
because my balance is back and my brain is in perfect working
order. I am passionate about understanding not only this time of
life, but also what this passage can bring to us emotionally, physically, and spiritually.

This is a tremendous time to be alive. Menopause does not have
to be the shameful, icky experience we have all anticipated. Once
again we baby boomers have decided not to take this thing sitting
down. We have never done this before, and now is not the time to
quit. We are still vital and energetic, but coming to terms with the
hormone mystery allows us to go out and truly enjoy this age. Balanced hormones coupled with wisdom is a lethal combination. The
only obstacle to experiencing all of our potential has been a lack
of understanding of the effects of hormone loss.

I do not in any way claim to know everything about hormones;
it is too big a subject, and new information comes out every week.
But I have opened the door. I have spent hundreds of hours
researching and meeting with professionals on the cutting edge. I
can hold my own with any doctor regarding this subject. Often I
am more informed, and that makes sense, because I have decided
to get to the bottom of my own hormonal mysteries. It has been
very empowering to understand the inner workings of my body. It
has helped me realize that there is cause and effect. If I choose to
ingest harmful foods, substances, and chemicals, I know there are
consequences. My body is so cleaned out of sugar that when I do
decide to indulge, I experience immediate consequences. My mood
changes, often I will get a yeast infection, and my energy drops. I
also know that it shoots my insulin levels way up, and that, in turn,
creates imbalances throughout my entire hormonal system.

One of the many blessings that has come from having lived with
cancer in my body is an appreciation of this complex and highly
sophisticated house in which I live and the thrill of being alive each
day. I wake up grateful. Every day is a borrowed one for me. It
doesn't matter if I live to be 105, my cancer taught me to be thank-

ful for all that is. I now treat my body with a tremendous amount of respect. Our bodies need to be well fed with delicious, beautifully prepared, *real* food. Our bodies need nourishment and proper rest. It took me a long time to understand the need to give my body a balanced amount of time out. It is something I am still working on; the workaholic in me is alive and well, but why wouldn't such a finely tuned machine need cooling out?

I used to take a weird kind of pleasure in outworking everyone. I am sure that the drive to push myself as hard as I have at times in my life comes from the child of the alcoholic in me, still trying to please that father. I now know that I am not invincible. In my frustration at not getting satisfactory medical answers to questions about the changes I was going through—physically, hormonally, and emotionally—I realized that it was up to me to do the work and learn how best to take care of myself. I couldn't find anyone to make sense of it for me, and this forced me to be proactive. This is what we all need to do. No one is going to do it for you! The women who look the best and feel the best are the ones who have pushed for more information. We're not at the top of the researchers' list. Only by yelling and screaming are they going to focus on our medical issues.

I know that in the coming years new and cutting-edge information on the hormonal system will become available, and I am going to be right there listening with an open mind, questioning and evaluating. I want to know what's new, and in turn I will pass on everything I learn about this subject to you. I love that I no longer sit in my doctor's office taking every answer and explanation at face value. I now question. I don't give up. Without this passion I would be a very unhappy woman right now. My menopausal symptoms were severe. My life had lost its quality, and for a time I thought that this was the way I was going to be—itchy, bitchy, sweaty, sleepy, bloated, forgetful, and all dried up: those seven miserable little menopause dwarfs. Add to that high insulin levels, and I was on a fast track to disease because of the departure of my hormones.

What a relief to understand that I am in control and have

enough information to know and feel when my finely tuned machine is out of whack. I can tell when it's even the tiniest bit off base. How empowering. When it's all working in concert, I feel like a living symphony. I experience joy and happiness that seem to want to burst out of me. I also feel proud to have this knowledge, so that I am not dependent upon anyone or anything telling me what I should do about my body. I know it's entirely up to me to care and protect this magnificent house I get to live in as if it were the most exquisite piece of art.

Hormones *are* the least understood medical mystery. We were never expected to live this long, so generations before us didn't get too worked up over this passage. With the loss of hormones, women contracted the diseases of aging and then died early. In those days, sixty, fifty, even forty was not considered too young to die. Aren't you shocked these days when someone that "young" dies? Medical technology has made tremendous strides. They have figured out how to keep us alive longer than ever before. We are going to live to be ninety or a hundred. But technology has not figured out how to ensure that these extra twenty or twenty-five years are quality ones. I don't know about you, but I want to be dancing on my one-hundredth birthday. Why not? With the new understanding of our hormones, it is possible to stay vital right up to the end. It is hard work, but once you understand, it becomes second nature. Unless I was starving to death, I would rather not eat than ingest fake food loaded with chemicals and preservatives.

But there is more to it. We are, as stated by the professionals and the wonderful, generous people I have talked with for this book, body, mind, and spirit. It's the whole package. Our job in life is to work on ourselves to become the best that we can be. Respecting our bodies is a vital component in our evolution, but evolving and growing emotionally and spiritually completes this trilogy. It is easy to become bitter and angry at what we didn't get; it is easy to blame others for what didn't work out in this life. True growth comes from seeing the part each of us has played in the drama of our individual lives. When we are able to see how we have contributed to those things that have brought us unhappiness or dissatisfaction, we can become accountable. Accountability is taking responsibility for the situation. Accountability is maturity as well as growth, and through this growth we can find resolution. It allows the situation to be rectified. Then each of us will be able to make corrections, or fix what is broken in our selves or our relationships, or make amends, or humble ourselves to do our part in reversing any negative energy that circles around us. It's an opportunity to apologize, to end all disagreements. Doing these things can free you and allow you to have the happiness you want at this age.

And then there is accountability to yourself. Are you pleased with who you are? If not, you can change. This is the spirit. Every day ask yourself, How can I become a better person? If you ask for it, it will come to you. We already have the answers within; it is up to each one of us to find them. It is my hope that this book has assisted you in your search. Just remember, you are a beautiful and magnificent person. This passage is your opportunity; this search for knowledge will open doors to rooms you never thought of entering. This is your time to soar, not those angst-filled years of youth. The time is now. The world is yours. You are at the top of your game. You have wisdom and perspective. Use it well, and pass it on to the next generation. We are here to help one another become all that we are capable of being. Turn on your personal light as bright as you can make it. The knowledge and wisdom you have gained will make you sexier. Because after all, we now know that these are *"the sexy years."*

RESOURCES

NATURAL HORMONE REPLACEMENT THERAPY

Dr. David Allen, M.D.
2211 Corinth Avenue, Suite 204
Los Angeles, CA 90064
(310) 966-9194

American Academy of Anti-Aging Medicine
1510 West Montana Street
Chicago, IL 60614
(773) 528-4333
www.worldhealth.net

Contact the academy to learn more about natural hormone replacement therapy. It is the leading organization of its kind, dedicated to the advancement of all therapeutic approaches that play a role in antiaging medicine, including natural bioidentical HRT.

Jennifer Berman, M.D.
Female Sexual Medicine Center at UCLA
924 Westwood Boulevard, Suite 515
Los Angeles, CA 90024
(310) 794-3030
(866) 439-2835
www.urology.medsch.ucla.edu/fsmc-jberman.html

Laura Berman, Ph.D.
Berman Center
211 East Ontario Street
Chicago, IL 60611
(800) 709-4709
www.bermancenter.com

Network for Excellence in Women's Sexual Health
www.newshe.com

Newshe is the official Web site of Drs. Laura and Jennifer Berman.

Joe Filbeck, M.D.
The Palm La Jolla Medical Spa
4510 Executive Drive, Suite 125
San Diego, CA 92121
(858) 457-5700
www.palmlajolla.com

Dr. Filbeck specializes in quality of life and antiaging medicine.

Michael Galitzer, M.D.
12381 Wilshire Boulevard, Suite 102
Los Angeles, CA 90025
(310) 820-6042
www.ahealth.com

Dr. Galitzer specializes in antiaging and natural bioidentical hormone replacement therapy.

Robert Greene, M.D.
1255 East Street, Suite 201
Redding, CA 96001
(530) 244-9052
www.specialtycare4women.com

Dr. Greene specializes in natural bioidentical hormone replacement therapy.

Prudence Hall, M.D.
1148 4th Street
Santa Monica, CA 90403
(310) 458-7979
(800) 442-4517
www.thehallcenter.com

Dr. Daniela Paunesky
3400 Old Milton Parkway
Bldg. C, Suite 380
Alpharetta, GA 30005
(770) 777-7707 Phone
(770) 777-7789 Fax
www.atlantaantiaging.com

Uzzi Reiss, M.D.
414 North Camden Drive, Suite 750
Beverly Hills, CA 90210
(310) 247-1300
www.uzzireissmd.com

Dr. Reiss, an ob/gyn, specializes in natural bioidentical hormone replacement therapy.

Dr. Diana Schwarzbein
5901 Encina Road, Suite A
Goleta, CA 93117
(805) 681-0003
www.drhormone.com

Dr. Schwarzbein is an endocrinologist who specializes in menopause and a pioneer in natural bioidentical hormone replacement therapy.

Eugene Shippen, M.D.
9 East Lancaster Avenue
Shillington, PA 19607
(610) 777-7896

Dr. Shippen specializes in male menopause (andropause).

Dr. Larry Webster
620 South Elm Street, Suite 312
Greensboro, NC 27406
(866) 266-8869

www.suzannesomers.com

My Web site has a link to information on bioidentical hormone replacement, including a reprint of the Women's Health Initiative Study.

American College for Advancement in Medicine (ACAM)
23121 Verdugo Drive, Suite 204
Laguna Hills, CA 92653
(800) 532-3688
www.acam.org

ACAM is dedicated to establishing certification and standards of practice or preventive medicine and the ACAM protocol.

American Health Institute
12381 Wilshire Boulevard
Los Angeles, CA 90025
(800) 392-2623
www.ahealth.com

Cofounded by Dr. Michael Galitzer, the institute is a pioneering research organization in the field of longevity medicine and the use of natural hormone replacement therapy.

WEB SITES FOR SEXUAL AIDS

www.goodvibes.com
www.grandopening.com

TESTING HORMONE LEVELS

Aeron LifeCycles
1933 Davis Street, Suite 310
San Leandro, CA 94577
(800) 631-7900
www.aeron.com

Sabre Sciences, Inc.
910 Hampshire Road, Suite P
Westlake Village, CA 91361
(888) 490-7300
www.sabresciences.com

COMPOUNDING PHARMACIES

ApothéCure, Inc.
4001 McEwen Road, Suite 100
Dallas, TX 75244
(972) 960-6601
(800) 969-6601
www.apothecure.com

The Compounding Pharmacy of Beverly Hills
9629 West Olympic Boulevard
Beverly Hills, CA 90212
(310) 284-8675
(888) 799-0212
www.compounding-expert.com

Health Pharmacies
2809 Fish Hatchery Road, Suite 103
Madison, WI 51713
(800) 373-6704

International Academy of Compounding Pharmacists
P.O. Box 1365
Sugar Land, TX 77487
(800) 927-4227
www.iacprx.org

You may call them or go to their Web site and enter your zip code
for a referral to the closest compounding pharmacy in your area.

Kronos Pharmacy
3675 South Rainbow Boulevard
Las Vegas, NV 89103
(800) 723-7455

Solutions Pharmacy
4632 Highway 58 North
Chattanooga, TN 37416
(423) 894-3222
(800) 523-1486
www.lakesidepharmacy.com/index2.ivnu

Steven's Pharmacy
1525 Mesa Verde Drive East
Costa Mesa, CA 92626
(800) 352-DRUG
www.stevensrx.com

Town Center Drugs and Compounding Pharmacy
72840 Highway 111
Westfield Shopping Town
Palm Desert, CA 92260
(760) 341-3984
(877) 340-5922

Women's International Pharmacy
12012 N. 111th Avenue
Youngtown, AZ 85363

2 Marsh Court
Madison, WI 53718
(800) 279-5708
www.womensinternational.com

RECOMMENDED READING

These books have assisted me in my journey to understand this difficult and complex passage and helped me in putting together *The Sexy Years.*

Berman, Jennifer, M.D., and Laura Berman, Ph.D. *For Women Only: A Revolutionary Guide to Overcoming Sexual Dysfunction and Reclaiming Your Sex Life.* New York: Holt, 2001.

Colgan, Michael. *Hormonal Health.* Vancouver, B.C.: Apple Publishing, 1996.

Collins, Joseph, N.D. *What's Your Menopause Type?* Roseville, Calif.: Prima Health, 2000.

Gershon, Michael D., M.D. *The Second Brain.* New York: Harper-Collins, 1998.

Hanley, Jesse Lynn, M.D., and Nancy Deville. *Tired of Being Tired.* New York: Putnam, 2001.

Lee, John R., M.D., with Virginia Hopkins. *What Your Doctor May Not Tell You About Menopause.* New York: Warner Books, 1996.

Lee, John R., M.D., with Jesse Hanley, M.D., and Virginia Hopkins. *What Your Doctor May Not Tell You About Premenopause.* New York: Warner Books, 1999.

Nelson, Miriam E., Ph.D., with Sarah Wernick, Ph.D. *Strong Women, Strong Bones.* New York: Perigee, 2000.

Regelson, William, M.D., and Carol Colman. *The Super-Hormone Promise: Nature's Antidote to Aging*. New York: Simon & Schuster, 1996.

Reiss, Uzzi, M.D., with Martin Zucker. *Natural Hormone Balance for Women*. New York: Pocket Books Health, 2001.

Sapolsky, Robert M. *The Trouble with Testosterone*. New York: Scribner, 1997.

Schwarzbein, Diana, M.D., and Nancy Deville. *The Schwarzbein Principle*. Health Communications, 1999.

Schwarzbein, Diana, M.D., with Marilyn Brown. *The Schwarzbein Principle II*. Health Communications, 2002.

Shippen, Eugene, M.D., and William Fryer. *The Testosterone Syndrome*. New York: M. Evans, 1998.

INDEX

Suzanne Somers'

slim
AND
sexy
forever

THE HORMONE SOLUTION FOR PERMANENT WEIGHT LOSS
AND OPTIMAL LIVING

SUZANNE SOMERS SHARES THE SECRET TO HER
FOUNTAIN OF YOUTH BY COMBINING HER EVER-
POPULAR SOMERSIZE SERIES WITH HER PHENOME-
NALLY SUCCESSFUL THE SEXY YEARS TO TEACH
READERS THE EASY AND EFFECTIVE WAY TO LOSE
WEIGHT, KEEP IT OFF FOR GOOD, AND BALANCE
HORMONES FOR OPTIMAL HEALTH AND VITALITY.

1-4000-5325-0

$25.95 Hardcover

WHEREVER BOOKS ARE SOLD
CROWN PUBLISHERS
CROWNPUBLISHING.COM